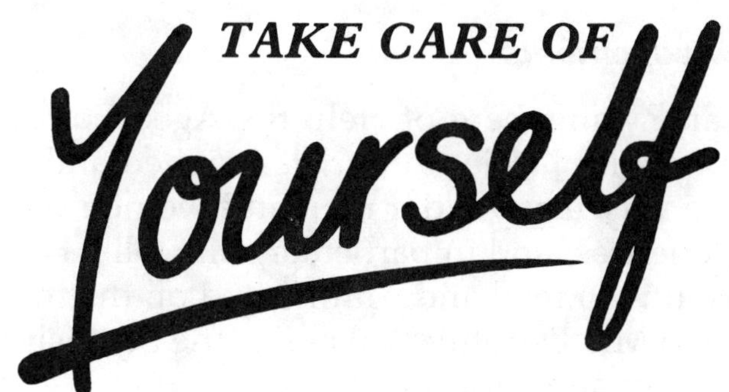

TAKE CARE OF *Yourself*

Help the Aged

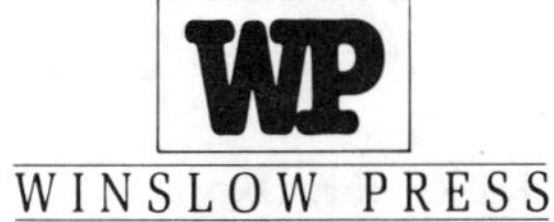

WINSLOW PRESS

Acknowledgements

Fiona van Zwanenberg of Help the Aged Education & Research Department who, with Jackie Corder, researched and wrote this book wishes to thank the very many older men and women who contributed their ideas and experiences; and in particular, Mrs Ollie Hollingsworth and Dr Keith Thompson who read and commented on the manuscript. Our thanks are also due to Mrs Dorothy Walster of the Scottish Health Education Group for her advice and support.

Help the Aged is a national charity dedicated to improving the quality of life of elderly people in need of help in the UK and overseas. We pursue this aim by raising and granting funds towards community-based projects, housing and overseas aid.

The **Scottish Health Education Group** promotes good health throughout Scotland. One special area of concern is action for health in later life.

Jointly published in 1988 by
Winslow Press, Telford Road, Bicester, Oxon OX6 0TS
and
Help the Aged, St James's Walk, London EC1R 0BE

Reprinted 1988

ISBN 0 86388 058 4

Phototypeset by Gecko Ltd, Bicester, Oxon

WP308/Printed in Great Britain by Oxford University Press

CONTENTS

Foreword

by

Sir Ferguson Anderson

OBE, KStJ, MD, FRCP

With the hindsight of experience advice regarding health care should have been an essential ingredient before the inception of the National Health Service. The publication of this handbook on how to look after oneself as age increases has now filled this gap in necessary information. This wide-ranging review of the changes to be expected with the process of ageing associated with a description of some common illnesses is written in simple, easy to understand language. Important aspects of physical, mental and social well-being are brought to attention and like most good maintenance manuals information is provided in detail of how to solve the particular cause of anxiety and where to get help.

Advice on how to keep fit physically and mentally is given covering topics such as exercise, education, personal appearance and travel. The aim is to encourage the achievement of a high quality of life even into extreme old age.

The fundamental truth that old age is not a disease is stressed and the supreme importance of a correct diagnosis when illness occurs is clearly stated.

This practical and interesting book will help many older people to take charge of their own life and enjoy it as they reap the reward of living in good health much longer than they expected.

Ferguson Anderson

INTRODUCTION

This book is about looking after yourself as you grow older. There are many guides to taking care of a frail older person, this is one for older people themselves.

In Chapter one, *Changes*, we look at the normal ageing process and some of the changes it can bring in a person's life. How do ordinary men and women cope with these when they occur and can their experience help others to deal with similar situations?

Chapter two, *Alone or Lonely*, recognises that one in three older people now live alone. Although many people lead contented solitary lives, living alone can be stressful, even when you are fit and well and have friends and a useful occupation. Being alone when ill or isolated from others can mean being lonely. Chapter two encourages you to take care of yourself and to reach out towards other people, especially those who may themselves be isolated. There are practical suggestions for making friends and coping with the particular loneliness that follows the loss of a loved partner.

Chapter three, *You and the system: Who helps?*, explains the range of care provided by The National Health Services, Social Services and some voluntary agencies. It helps you to get the best from the system and contains useful hints on subjects such as dealing with your doctor, going into hospital or finding help to care for a relative.

Chapter four, *Mobility*, is about the pace of life in later years. Many of the older
men and women whose opinions helped us create this book felt that ageing, for them, meant slowing down but an equal number told us that they were busier and more outgoing in retirement than ever before in their lives. Chapter four is about achieving a good quality of life, even if it is lived at a slower pace. There is practical advice about keeping active and mobile and about making sure that your mind, as well as your body, is in good shape.

Chapter five, *Very Senior Citizens — Just for You*, was contributed for us by an author who is herself 98 years old. Mrs Dorothy Moriarty lives in a RUKBA Old Peoples' home in Camberley. Help the Aged counts it a privilege to publish her personal account of growing old. Her courage and good sense are an inspiration to us all.

In addition to our thanks to Mrs Moriarty, Help the Aged would like to thank the scores of older men and women who wrote to us with their ideas about health, while we were researching this book. Their help has meant that we can offer the best kind of advice — advice based on experience.

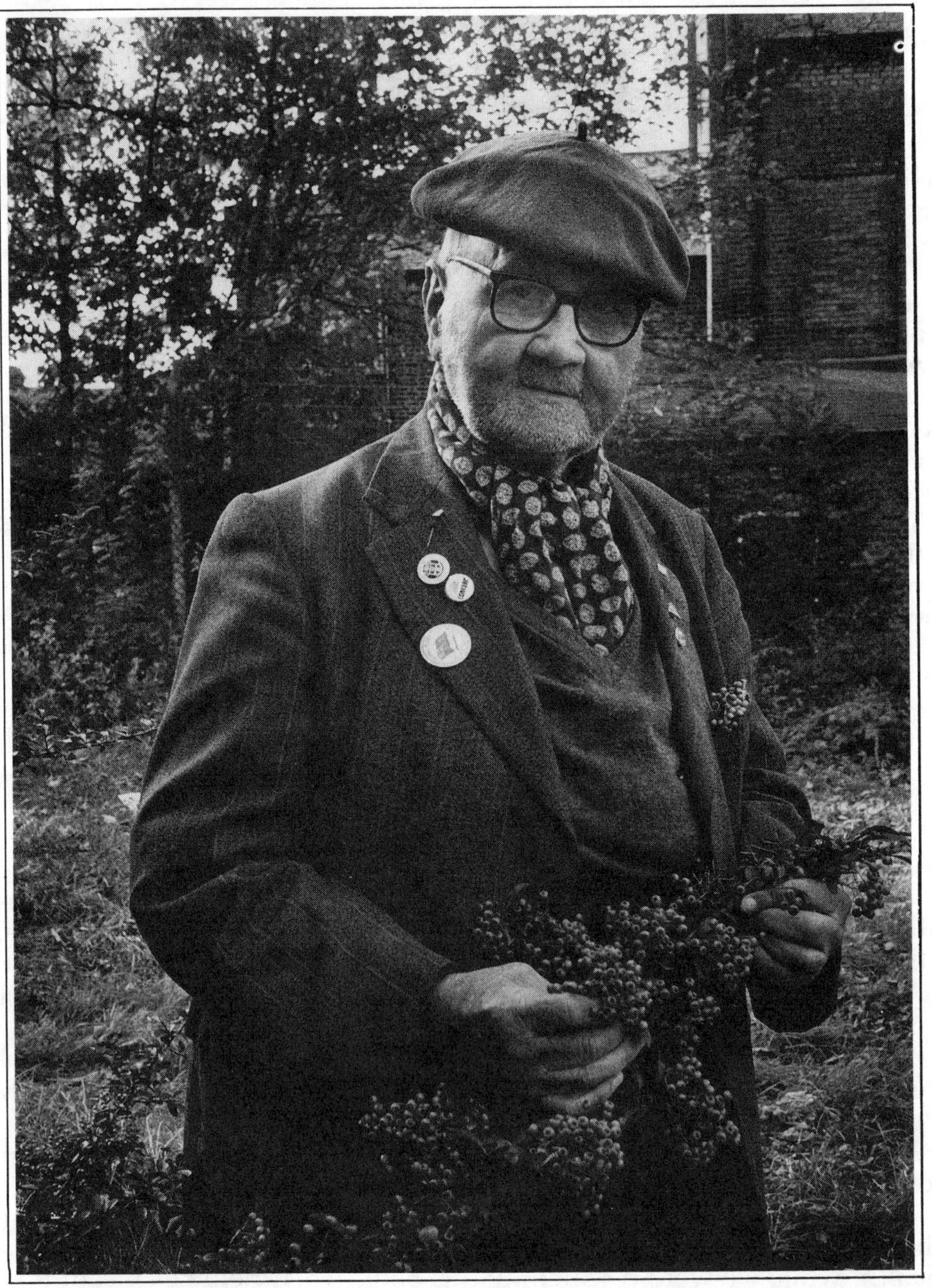

1

CHANGES

"I knew I was old when . . ."

"I think we've got to accept when we're getting older and we've got to be prepared to slow down and realise that we can't do today what we did ten years ago."

"You most likely do everything you did, with the exception of really physical exercise, but you do it slower and you take longer to do it."

During 1984, men and women over seventy in different parts of the country came together in groups to discuss health topics. All of them said that same kind of thing when asked what ageing meant to them.

". . . slowing down."

". . . slowing up."

". . . not being able to do what you used to do."

But they also described feeling just the same 'inside' as when they were much younger.

"I don't feel as though I've aged."

"I feel no different whatsoever from when I was 14."

"I don't feel my age . . . I don't feel like I expected."

"I'm bound to be old if I'm 74. But the thing is I don't feel that I'm old."

For most of us, ageing is a gradual process, but some sudden event, or a comment made by a friend or relative, can bring it home to you with a sudden shock.

Sometimes it can be an amusing situation although you might not see the funny side until afterwards. One older man described how he knelt down to peer under a gas fire and found he had stuck fast. His eight stone wife had to fetch a neighbour and it took their combined efforts to help him get up.

Hearing a child being told to give up a seat for 'the old man' or 'that old lady' and realising that they mean you, can come as a shock, as can an unexpected glimpse of yourself in a mirrored shop window or doorway. The grey-haired, elderly figure may be quite different to the picture you have of yourself.

What changes ought you to expect as you grow older?

Some physical and mental changes happen to everyone as they age. Some things, like increasing long-sightedness or going bald cannot be controlled. Others, such as becoming overweight (the so-called 'middle-aged spread') need not happen and can be reversed. It is important to realise that ageing is not in itself a disease, and that any illness or complaint should never be dismissed as 'just old age'. Any physical or psychological changes should not be ignored; the sooner you see your doctor, the better the chance that you will be cured.

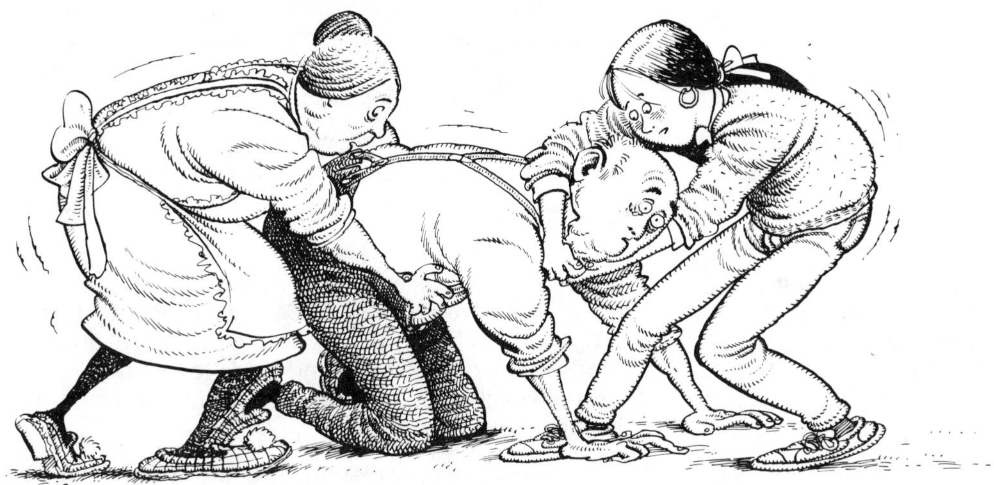

Some changes of normal ageing and what you can do about them

CHANGES	ACTION
Eyesight	
The lens of the eye often becomes less elastic as you age and begins to harden. It may take on a yellowish tinge which affects your ability to distinguish colours.	Make sure you have regular check-ups and that your glasses are still suitable.
The lens may also become less able to change focus, leading to long-sightedness. Many people in their late forties need reading glasses except in bright light.	Is your lighting at home as good as it should be? Check stairs and landings are clearly lit, and that there are no gloomy corners. This is particularly important if you regularly have to get up during the night.

Hearing

Many people notice some hearing loss by the age of 50. In many cases, this change is brought about by environment and not simply through ageing. Sometimes, where a person has worked for years in a noisy environment, hearing may be damaged. Injuries and accidents can also cause hearing loss.

Noticeable dulling of hearing can be due to something as simple as a build-up of wax in the ears.

Hearing aids are often a great help; however it does take time to adjust to them. They amplify all sounds and therefore it may be difficult to distinguish conversation from background noise. Having lived in a relatively silent world for some time, the wearer should use the aid only for short periods initially and practise conversation in a room with little background noise. The NHS provide models free of charge; there are a wide selection available. If you are thinking of purchasing one commercially make sure it is suitable for your type of hearing loss.

Never poke anything into your ears — have them syringed by a nurse or other qualified person.

Skin

All skin becomes less elastic as it grows older, because of loss of subcutaneous fat. Skin also changes in appearance, because of changes in pigment and damage to tiny veins.

Sunshine is a vital source of vitamin D. This is essential to prevent loss of Calcium in ageing. Lying around in the full sun for very long periods of time tends to dry out the skin, and leads to ageing. Benefits of the sun can be enjoyed by using cream to protect the skin.

Bathing can be very pleasurable and relaxing, the use of bath oil enhances the experience. Too many long, hot baths can dry out the skin; however, showers are an alternative.

Taste

If you have ever said that food doesn't taste as good as it used to, the reason is probably to be found in your mouth rather than because of changes in farming methods. The number of taste buds on your tongue decreases as you get older, and by the late seventies and eighties most people have lost 80% of their ability to taste different flavours.

There is nothing you can do to preserve your sense of taste. However, the flavour of food can be enhanced by the use of onions, peppers, garlic and spices. **Do avoid the temptation to add lots of salt to your food to increase flavour.** Doctors now agree that we should cut down on the amount of salt we add to our food, and try to eat plenty of fresh fruit and vegetables.

Hair

Grey hair is hair which lacks the pigment which gives hair its colour — blonde, black or brunette. Most people have some grey in their hair by their mid-forties, and practically everyone in their seventies has grey or white hair.

Some people find that their hair becomes thinner as they grow older. Our hair is constantly being renewed throughout life and the rate of re-growth may slow as we get older.

Baldness, which is much more common in men than in women, is an inherited trait and so far is irreversible. True baldness should not be confused with temporary hair loss due to an illness, which can occur during the menopause.

Mrs Hollingsworth, who is in her eighties, offers a practical suggestion: "I've bought a very nice wig which is always ready to put on should I get asked out and I can't get to a hairdresser. I always feel better if my hair isn't looking a sight". Other people choose to have their hair dyed, or to simply leave it its natural grey colour. It can look very distinguished and elegant.

There is a place for 'grey pride', where a grey or white head is respected as a badge of experience and wisdom.

Think about how long it is since you last changed your hair-style — you might consider asking a young relative for advice. Teenagers can be remarkably sensitive and helpful. After all, they themselves care very much about appearances and are usually very much in touch with fashions.

A person who is bald or who has thin hair may find it helpful to cover their head in cold weather, as they may experience greater heat loss during this time. They should also be careful not to get too much sun on the scalp during the summer months.

Teeth

In Britain, 75% of all men and women have lost all their teeth by the time they are 75. The cause is not a natural ageing process. Tooth loss is due to a diet which contains too much sugar, gum disease and inadequate quantities of fluoride in drinking water.

After the age of 40, extractions are much more likely to be due to gum disease than to decay.

Regular brushing with a toothpaste containing fluoride will prevent the build up of plaque which causes tooth decay. The use of dental floss is also a very effective way to control gum disease.

Hard, calcified plaque, called **calculus** is the main cause of gum disease. Your dentist or a dental hygienist can remove these deposits and regular brushing using a small-headed soft brush will keep your gums healthy.

If you have dentures, do wear them. Your gums can shrink if you leave uncomfortable dentures out. Painful, ill-fitting, dentures are unnecessary. Get professional advice.

It is important to realise that some people of 100 years still have all their own teeth!

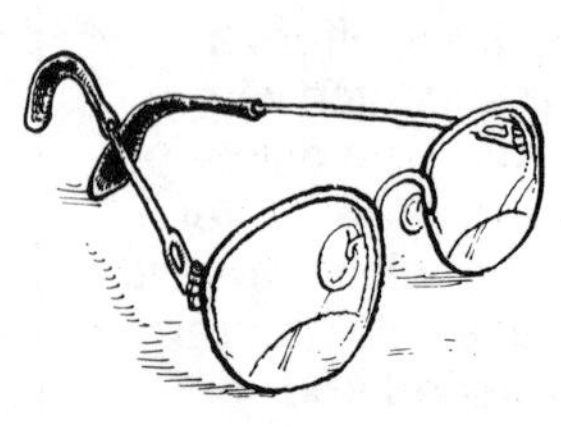

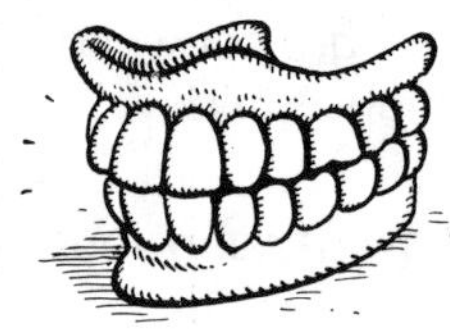

If you think about spectacles, some degree of deafness, skin changes, grey hair and false teeth, it can add up to a pretty depressing picture, but there is no need to let this image lower your spirits. None of these need interrupt an active and enjoyable way of life.

Most older people are in good health and actively enjoy life. They are often far more contented and satisfied with their lives than their middle-aged relatives.

"I certainly think it's one of the happiest times of my life — much happier than when I was a youngster."

"One of the good things about this age is that you, having had responsibilities all of your life, then throw them away and you remake your own programme and I find that quite a release . . . release from strict routine and timetabling . . . to be free to choose what I want to do on a particular day instead of having to get dressed up for 8 o'clock every morning and be on parade all day."

"You can do as you like, you can go where you like as long as your health's OK."

Watch points

There are some conditions which can occur as you age which are not part of normal ageing, but which may be overlooked. We are all guilty of thinking 'it's just old age' when the condition is a disease and **treatable**.

Abnormal changes in the eyes are a particular example.

CATARACT — This is a clouding of the lens of the eye, which blocks or changes the amount of light needed for vision. Poor vision may lead people to give up driving.	Over 95% of operations to remove a cataract are successful, bringing a great transformation in a person's life. Many old people need not lose their licence: all that may be necessary is a change of glasses.
GLAUCOMA is a particular eye problem which is fairly common in later life. It arises when there is an abnormally high fluid pressure within the eye. If untreated it can eventually lead to blindness.	Glaucoma is easily detected. You should report symptoms such as blurred vision, painful watering eyes and headache. An annual eye check-up by a qualified ophthalmologist or optician will detect early symptoms, and the condition can be easily treated at an early stage.

Mental changes

Physical change in a person may be obvious but some people worry needlessly about changes which are **not** so visible — mental changes. The fear of becoming 'senile' causes unnecessary anxiety for many people, despite the fact that 80% of men and women over 80 show no evidence of such change.

What are the facts about mental changes in later life?

Intelligence

Intelligence, like other human capacities such as height and strength, continues to grow until somewhere between 15 and 25 years of age. Although intellectual capacity definitely stops growing, we don't stop learning in our late teens or early twenties. Intellectual capacity is in any case not the same as intellectual achievement or wisdom. These continue to grow, affected by experience, technical skill and personal aptitudes.

We do know that some older people may show a decline in intellectual capacity where they are asked to:

► acquire new concepts;
► apply existing knowledge quickly and accurately to complicated situations.

This is because they have to unlearn before learning again. Most younger people find this easier.

We all know some older people who have impaired short-term memory. But there seems to be evidence that practice helps. In the same way as regular physical exercise keeps your body supple, mental exercise can help overcome memory failures. As they say, 'If you don't use it you lose it'. In fact, it does seem that in many cases memory failures arise because the person is not sufficiently interested to keep trivial events in mind.

Most of us develop our own tricks to jog memory, such as linking a name with a descriptive phrase.

'Mr Walker, a great talker' or developing rituals: 'The greenhouse key **always** goes in the top drawer in the kitchen.' But we shouldn't be in too much of a hurry to blame momentary memory lapses on old age. Almost everyone forgets names, appointments, routes — but a twenty-five-year old who can't remember where he left his car in a multi-storey car park doesn't automatically assume that he's becoming senile. Nor does the thirty-five-year-old mother resolutely refusing to learn anything about her son's home computer believe that she **can't** master this information. She merely chooses not to try.

We should beware of selling older people short when we take it for granted that their intellectual capacity is less than that of the young. Eric Midwinter, in a recent book, pointed out some factors to bear in mind.

▶ Most intelligence tests were designed for children, whereas adults bring their experience and greater sophistication to the problem. They may be irritated and frustrated by a problem to which a child would happily offer the 'correct' solution.

▶ If we compare older people with younger people in their twenties and thirties, we must also compare their different educational experiences. The older group may have had scant educational opportunities and their different scores will reflect this. If a man of seventy does not do as well as one of twenty, we are not entitled to assume that his intelligence has declined since he himself was twenty years old.

▶ People's general health and morale affect their performance in tests. This may seem very obvious, but it is particularly important with older people. If you are frail, have problems with eyesight and hearing and are anxious and worried about being tested you will not be likely to do as well as you might. Also, if you've been told that you're 'past it' and feel unconfident about your own ability, you're not going to be able to compete on an equal footing with a cheerful, confident youngster.

One in twenty of the students registered for courses at The Open University is over 60, and a study has been made of the needs, attitudes and experiences of this group of older students. When their performance overall was compared with that of younger students it was found that the older group did much better than the under-60s in the middle range of scores (40%–69%) and fewer of them did either very well or very badly.

Examinations did seem to be particularly stressful for the older students, however, and they did much better on continuous assessment than in the formal three-hour examinations. As one older student explained:

"I have particular difficulty in recalling what I have learned. I particularly notice this in exams, when facts that I should have at my fingertips elude me until the exam is over and then come flooding in."

Despite such difficulties, the study concluded that older people were 'stimulated and refreshed' by taking part in a course of study and needed no special arrangements to be made on their behalf — that they could compete on equal terms with students of their children's and grandchildren's age.

Normal mental changes in later life do not, in fact, amount to a great problem. Few of us are asked to operate at the limits of our intellectual capacity in situations of great importance during our ordinary, everyday lives. Normal ageing need hold no fears.

But people **are** afraid of **abnormal** ageing, of brain failure. What are the facts about this?

First of all, mental confusion is not a sign of normal ageing. Very often confusion is a symptom of an illness, or it may be due to side-effects of a drug. Both these situations are temporary and reversible.

Depression in an older person can also be confused with dementia. An unhappy, depressed person, who is perhaps isolated after a bereavement, can show symptoms which appear very much like those of dementia. However, with skilled assessment and treatment, a depressed older person has the same chance of recovery as a younger patient. In times of stress, such as moving home, going into hospital and, most of all, bereavement, we are all susceptible to feelings of confusion or gloominess. With the right sort of support, however, these feelings can be overcome.

Nonetheless, a minority of old people, particularly those over 80, do suffer from brain failure.

Dementia

When a person has dementia there is declining mental capacity due to an abnormal loss of brain cells. It is permanent and irreversible and tends to get worse. The most common form of this brain failure is called **Alzheimer's disease**.

There is another fairly common form of dementia which occurs more often in older men than women. It is called **arteriosclerotic dementia** and it is caused by narrowing arteries in the brain which cut off the blood supply and cause groups of brain cells to die.

If a person has severe dementia it can mean a heavy burden of worry and responsibility for the family and particularly the husband or wife.

Changes of personality are often the most distressing symptom of this disease. A quiet, reserved person may become boisterous and aggressive and perhaps use violent or obscene language.

Memory loss, wandering, not knowing where they are and perhaps trying to find an old home or long-dead family members can create problems in the home environment.

Do ask for help if you are having problems in coping with a dementia sufferer. There is respite available, through day hospitals, day care centres, sitting-in services etc. Ask your GP, health visitor or social worker or contact your local Age Concern office.

Sudden changes

So far, we have talked about changes which may creep up on you gradually. But sometimes a change can come with devastating suddenness; literally at a stroke.

Strokes

Stroke is mainly a disease of later life, although younger people are affected too. A stroke is caused by an interruption of the blood supply to part of the brain. A gradual narrowing of the blood vessel occurs before the stroke. The side of the body which is damaged in a stroke is opposite to the side of the brain which has been damaged. This is because the nerves in the brain which control movement and sensation cross over to supply the other side of the body. Damage to the left side of the brain produces most effects on the right side of the body and vice versa. As the speech centre is in the left side of the brain, damage on that side is most likely to affect speech. Stroke is an illness which is very much feared and fears are fed by all sorts of myths which surround it. For example, there is a common, but totally false belief that a third stroke is always fatal. Obviously some people do die of strokes. But recovery **is** possible and many people have fought back to a normal life after a disabling illness.

Miss Cummings is a single woman who worked in her local library for most of her life. She had previously cared for both her parents during their final years and, having retired at sixty, was enjoying her independence and leisure to follow new pursuits and interests. However, a few days before her 65th birthday, she had a severe stroke. She described what happened:

"I lost the use of my right leg and my right arm and lost my speech. The doctors and nurses and a blind physiotherapist were all very kind. My speech very slowly came back and the use of my right leg. I am sorry to say that my temper was not so good in that first year. However, after that first year I pulled myself together. I first tried to knit (no use), then I started to crochet quite successfully and made several things . . . I read and write my own poetry, and sing. After 15 years I manage very well and keep very happy. I have had to learn to write with my left hand. I keep very happy and also my memory is very good."

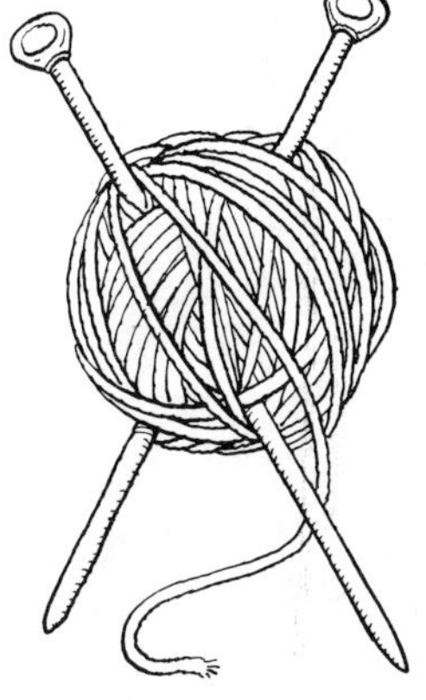

Can you do anything to avoid a stroke?

▶ Some strokes can be prevented if high blood pressure is detected and treated.

▶ Eating large amounts of salt is now known to be a factor in high blood pressure. Ought you to cut down?

▶ Heavy drinking also increases the risk of a stroke, because of its link with high blood pressure. A safe level of drink is up to 13 standard drinks per week for women and up to 20 standard drinks per week for men, provided it is spread over the week. A standard drink is half a pint of beer or lager, a glass of table wine or a standard pub measure of spirits. However, it should be stressed that drinking within these limits may still lead to confusion and accidents. Any drinking bout can be dangerous, particularly to people who are already a little unsteady on their feet.

Self-help

The Chest, Heart and Stroke Association began a volunteer stroke scheme in the late 70s, to help people recover from a stroke. One of the most upsetting and frustrating effects of a stroke is the total or partial loss of speech. The most severe effect in which the person loses the ability to form or understand words is called **aphasia**, but there can be a whole range of other, less drastic effects on language and speech.

Volunteers organised by The Chest, Heart and Stroke Association have so far helped more than 500 stroke patients through intensive, one to one, speech therapy, usually under the guidance of local doctors and speech therapists. They also run stroke clubs all over the country.

Stroke clubs vary enormously according to the needs of their users. Miss Irene Clegg has attended her nearest centre for nearly two years. She is confined to a wheelchair and depends on transport provided by her local Social Services Department to get to the club.

"It's my only regular outing," she said. "A lot of us here live alone and the club gives us a chance to meet people. We all understand what it feels like and we can help one another. Take Agnes, for instance; she's really improved since she started coming here. Her speech was very bad and she didn't want to try, but with us, she felt able to have a go. We know what it's like, you see."

If a close relative suffers a stroke, the problems for the rest of the family can be great. The patient will be frustrated by inability to do things previously taken for granted and may also become very depressed.

People who have recently had a stroke can seem very selfish, because they are involved with themselves, trying to come to terms with the changes that have overtaken them. This can be a painful experience. Miss Temple had lived an independent and active life and spoke bitterly about her experience to a visiting nurse:

"At 81 I had a stroke, and stayed in the hospital for one month and eventually went home. I can't do many things I used to do. My walking is a limp, my speech is slurred, I can no longer eat the food I want. I can no longer attend the activities I enjoyed or visit friends like I used to . . . I can no longer attend church activities, nor can I attend the chapel itself, I feel so depressed so many times, but I don't know why. The hours go so slow."

Someone who feels like this can receive help and comfort from sharing their experience with others who understand. This is one of the main benefits of a stroke club, as well as getting the person out of the house and providing an interest. It is a chance to talk to others who have experienced the same sort of problems as you have and to share ideas for coping with difficulties.

You can make contact with a stroke club by writing to:

The Chest, Heart and Stroke Association
Tavistock House North   or   65 North Castle Street
Tavistock Square   Edinburgh EH2 3LT
London WC1H 9JE

Heart disease

There is one major change in the human heart as it grows older which contributes to heart disease.

Atherosclerosis is a build-up of fatty material on the walls of the arteries, which makes them narrow and interferes with the flow of blood. It causes hardening and loss of elasticity in the arterial wall. This is rare before 30, but by 50 many people develop this condition.

Risk factors which can cause heart disease

► Eating too much food containing fats and sugar
► Being overweight
► Not getting enough exercise
► Not being able to relax, being overworked and under pressure
► Smoking cigarettes
► A high blood pressure
► Heredity — your family history

What can you do to avoid these risks, or reduce them as much as possible?

'Eating to your Heart's Content'

Diet plays an important part in the prevention and control of heart disease. We would all be healthier if we followed four main guidelines:
Eat more fibre (roughage, as it used to be called)
Eat less fat
Eat less sugar
Eat less salt
There is a useful booklet called *Beating Heart Disease* available free from the:

Health Education Authority
PO Box 413
London SE99 67E

Scottish Health Education Group (SHEG)
Health Education Centre
Woodburn House
Canaan Lane
Edinburgh EH10 4SG

Another helpful publication is *Eat to your Heart's Content* from SHEG.

Smoking

Whatever your age, giving up smoking cigarettes is the single most effective action you can take to improve your health. It is a myth that smoking doesn't matter if you've smoked all your life without any apparent ill effects.

For many of us, smoking is part and parcel of our daily lives. We might argue that, in later life, it provides 'one of our few remaining pleasures'. But we ought to know the facts:

▶ If you have had a heart attack, your chances of survival are improved if you give up smoking cigarettes.
▶ If you continue to smoke as you grow older, your chances of suffering from heart disease, lung cancer or bronchitis are increased.
▶ Smoking increases the chances of an infection becoming a serious illness.
▶ The effects of smoking lengthen the amount of time it takes you to get back to normal after an illness, particularly with chest infections, bronchitis and pneumonia.

Exercise

For many of us, exercise means keeping fit, but what is fitness?

Fitness is a measure of how effectively your body can respond to a sudden demand, such as hurrying to catch a bus. If an unplanned burst of activity leaves you gasping for breath and very aware of your heart pounding, then you're not very fit.

All of us have a **fitness gap**, the difference between our present state of fitness and our potential, the way we **could** be if we were at our best. For an athlete like Steve Cram, the gap is a tiny one and his best efforts could only produce a minute improvement in fitness. But for the ordinary, unfit majority, the good news is that we could reduce our **fitness gap** significantly. Because we're unfit, a programme of exercise will bring very great rewards. To find out more about exercise programmes and fitness, contact:

The Sports Council   Scottish Sports Council
16 Upper Woburn Place   1/3 St Colme Street
London WC1H 0QP   Edinburgh EH3 6AA

High blood pressure

Blood pressure is the pressure the heart applies to pump blood round the body. At times of stress, anger, fear or exertion, the blood flow is increased by the release of stress hormones. If the level is consistently high, even at a time of rest, this is known as **hypertension** and puts a strain on the heart. Stress and being unable to relax can be major causes of high blood pressure.

Arteriosclerosis and atherosclerosis can be associated with high blood pressure because the narrowed arteries make the heart work harder to pump the blood round the body.

Angina is caused by an inadequate blood supply to the heart during exercise. The symptoms are severe chest pain, dizziness and sickness and shortness of breath. It is usually relieved by rest.

Mrs Burrows, who has lived with angina attacks for some years, describes her experience:

"To manage the angina I have a home-help twice a week, exceptionally good, and a Batricar for mobility. About the house I do a little, try not to rush or become tense and keep away, if possible, from stressful situations. I try to keep to a sensible diet, plenty of fruit and vegetables, and keep occupied with 'sitting down' hobbies. Also I go out in the fresh air whenever possible."

Continence

In her book about the experience of growing old in Britain, Gladys Elder described her anguish when a bout of illness and the drugs she had been prescribed caused her to become incontinent.

"This, I decided, was the end. I would commit suicide . . . later it was discovered that one of the many tablets I'd been taking had caused the diarrhoea. If only they had told me at the time of this possibility, how much suffering I would have been saved."

Many older people share her despairing attitude — that incontinence is 'the last straw' — and fear that they will inevitably have to live with this distressing situation. Unfortunately, relatives and even doctors may share this hopeless attitude and will not encourage active treatment and self-help strategies. Don't let yourself **ever** be fobbed off by the attitude which explains an incontinence problem as 'just old age'.

Some facts

In some older people the capacity of the bladder may reduce from about a pint to about half a pint. So it is neither wrong nor unusual for those affected by this change to find that they need to go to the lavatory more frequently than when they were younger.

While incontinence is not unusual among elderly people (about 12% of women and about 8% of men over 65) it is by no means only older people who have this problem.

Incontinence is a symptom, like pain or fever, that something is wrong. Often it is a simple infection or a muscle weakness which can be treated successfully. Men who have trouble with their prostate gland may feel the urge to pass urine because the enlarged gland is putting pressure on the bladder or they may have problems with dribbling urine. For some women, who have weak pelvic floor muscles, which have usually been over-stretched in childbirth, any slight irritation or stress, such as a sneeze, leads to leakage of urine.

Exercises and a regular routine of toilet visits can help to maintain continence for both men and women.

What can you do to help yourself?

▶ **Pelvic floor exercises.** These can be practised at any time and in any position — lying in bed, sitting watching TV or standing at the sink. Tighten just the back passage muscles and then the front, and then both together. Count four slowly and then release. Do this four times, repeating the whole sequence every hour if possible.

▶ **Drink regularly** throughout the day, even if you're not thirsty. Up to 8 cups a day is a recommended amount. Restricting the amount you drink may make your urine strong and smelly. However, you may prefer not to drink so much in the late evening, as this can lead to the need to pass urine during the night.

▶ **Train yourself** to pass urine at regular intervals, eg. every two hours, whether or not you feel the urge.

Rheumatism and arthritis

Rheumatism is an everyday word which most of us use to describe various aches and pains.

Arthritis is a disease — it involves inflammation of a joint or joints. There are two main types of arthritis.

Osteoarthritis, sometimes known as osteorthrosis, is a joint disease in which there is erosion of the cartilage and thereafter damage to the underlying parts of the bones and joints. Osteoarthritis is normally put down to 'wear and tear' of the big joints, but can result from an injury (eg. footballer's knees).

Rheumatoid arthritis is a very different disease. The linings of the joints become inflamed. It usually attacks the small joints in the hands and feet. Rheumatoid arthritis is associated with general ill-health, and may affect other organs in the body. Anaemia and understandable depression can accompany this illness.

Arthritis can affect anyone at any age — about 7 million adults and children in Britain are estimated to suffer from rheumatic disease at any one time.

It should **never** be dismissed as 'just old age'. Research into causes and treatment is being carried out and there is optimism about finding a cure.

Treatment

Various treatments have been used to good effect. If you suffer from this disease you may well be offered:

▶ In the acute phase bed rest and gentle exercise in equal amounts. Hydrotherapy may help and swimming is one way in which this can be achieved;
▶ Splinting to prevent deformity during rest and exercises;
▶ Physiotherapy including hydrotherapy, heat treatment and massage;
▶ Diet — some people notice for themselves that certain foods make the arthritis worse;
▶ Surgery, eg. joint replacement;
▶ Drug treatment;
▶ Occupational therapy.

Advances in surgery and the development of artificial joints have brought relief to many. One man in his seventies who had developed a drink problem in the years preceding his hip replacement found that he saved the price of a bottle of whisky every week after his operation which had freed him from fairly constant pain!

To be considered for surgery you should be in good general health and ideally the damage should be limited to one or two joints. For some people, like Mrs Davison, a joint replacement has meant a new lease of life:

"The other day I went to a bazaar with stalls and a lady was behind one of them and she had crutches and she noticed my hands. I had arthritis and she had very bad knees, and a hospital wanted to replace the knee joints. She said she didn't think it was a successful operation so she wouldn't have it done. I told her different. Like her, I had always fought against it and carried on. Eight years ago my knees locked bent and I had the operation. It was wonderful to be able to stand up straight, but to walk again was marvellous!"

Sharing your experiences like Mrs Davison is what this book is about. As one older widow, talking of her husband's death, said to us: "Only those who know, know".

The discussion groups which met to talk about health were able to share their experiences with one another and to help each other to understand the changes which were happening to them in the later years of their lives. You also may find support and help from others in your situation and many day centres and clubs now run health courses which can help you to get the best out of your retirement years.

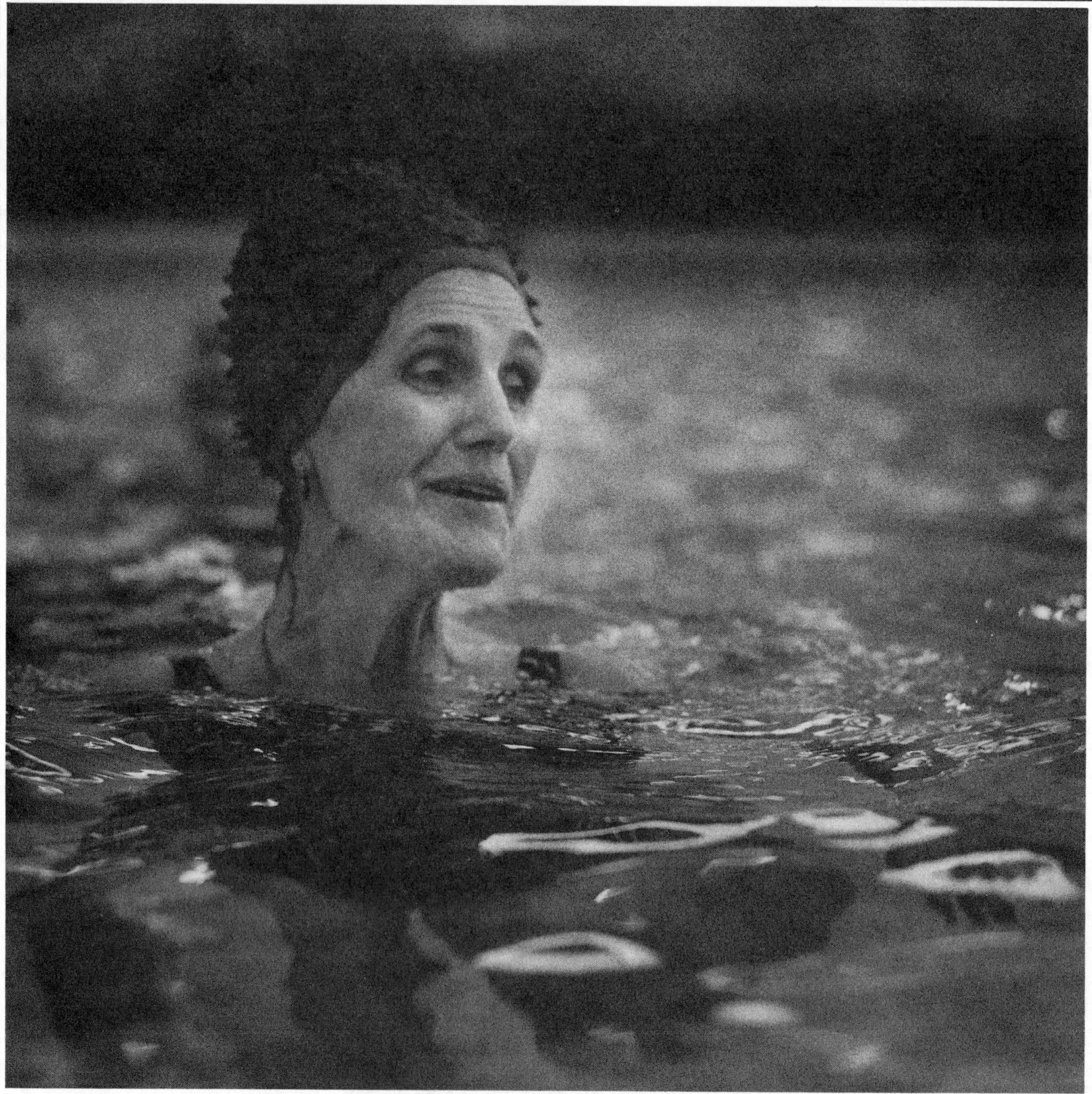

2

ALONE OR LONELY

One third of people of retirement age now live alone. Although there has been an increase in the proportion of young adults living by themselves, no other generation has such a high proportion of men and women, particularly women, living in rooms, flats and houses on their own.

Some live alone through choice — they are the natural 'loners' who have spent their entire adult lives on their own and who, in later life, simply continue with the habits of a lifetime. But for each person who chooses a single lifestyle, there are a great many who have had it thrust upon them.

Often being alone is due to bereavement, the loss of a marriage partner, a relative or friend or the loss of a job and the social contacts which went with going out to work.

Miss Wright and Miss Peasegood are examples of the first group, older women who have never married and have lived alone all their lives. They have both thought deeply about what is involved in living alone and have come to terms with it.

"I have always liked being independent and had no wish to marry. Were I married now, I should be a burden to my partner, which I should hate."
(*Miss Wright*)

"Living alone can be quite lonely; this can be relieved by being surrounded by kind, practical friends. A little more philosophy, if you wish to have friends you must be friendly, also to learn the art of giving as well as receiving."
(*Miss Peasegood*)

It would be foolish to pretend that some of the health problems faced by older people are not made worse by having to cope alone, by having "too much time to concentrate on oneself, and too little incentive to get on with things".

It can be a miserable and exhausting business struggling alone with the system, as Mrs Morris, a widow recently discharged from hospital, describes:

"When I came out of hospital, living alone, there was no help except a kind neighbour. Eventually as things got worse an old office friend offered to help with shopping and personal jobs. I managed for about six months, when finally I had to have the district nurse and she got in touch with the local Social Services Department and from them I obtained disabled items and an orange car badge and am now waiting for an allowance from the DHSS.

"I now cope much better and am not so bitter. I registered with a disabled magazine and have pen friends. I can do light gardening, but I have to have help with most jobs."

Retiring from work can present special problems for the person who lives alone. Often there is a decline in social life, which may have been founded on friendships with colleagues, whose interests no longer coincide. If retiring from work and perhaps being less mobile and having less money to spend on outings has meant a new problem of loneliness, it can best be tackled by having a close look at the situation.

Are there times when you feel particularly lonely and other times when you are quite happy to be on your own? Many people find public holidays and weekends, particularly Sundays, the worst. When are the good times, when don't you feel conscious of loneliness and isolation?

Can you devise ways of coping with the worst times, perhaps by putting off some activity until that time, inviting a visitor into your home or involving yourself in a new hobby?

Most of us feel much brighter once we've looked at a problem squarely and really considered how to deal with it.

If your loneliness comes from the death of a partner don't set yourself goals that are too ambitious. Someone recently bereaved is coping with major stress. It is no time to give yourself extra challenges to meet. It can take all your strength and resolution to pull your life together and find ways of carrying on.

Many people have commented on the help and support offered by relatives and friends at this time, and it is important not to reject this:

"The support of those around is a tremendous help and kindliness of folk is outstanding, and the many little ways people seek to help must never, never be spurned by too great independence; if the offer can be accepted grab it gratefully, little gifts and kindly words are offered with an overflowing heart."

(Mrs V J Sykes writing 18 months after the death of her husband.)

Taking charge of your life

Margaret Hall's husband died of cancer after a year-long battle which involved three operations, radiotherapy and chemotherapy.

After his death she was both physically and emotionally exhausted and in no state to make positive plans for a life on her own. But two years later, although she still missed him and probably always would do, she had made a determined effort to face up to living alone. 'You can try and be useful; it helps, even if your heart isn't really in it.'

Mrs Hall has a mentally handicapped grand-daughter and devotes a great deal of time to helping with her care. She has also found a full-time job for the summer months, as warden of the small farm caravan-site where she and her husband had kept their caravan for the past six years.

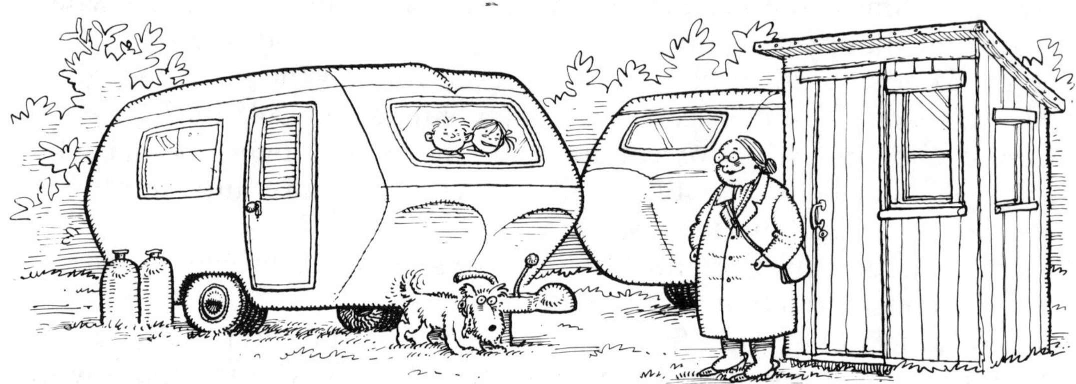

It can take courage to look for new ways of getting into company, when you are very sad and can't really be bothered, but the effort is worthwhile.

10 Ways of getting into company

1 Find a job
A little part-time job offers one of the best ways of meeting people — a friendly workplace provides an instant circle of contacts.

2 Help others out

Working alongside other like-minded people for a common cause is one of the easiest and most natural ways to make friends. Most voluntary organisations will welcome the help of people who can spare time and energy to help others.

3 Join a club

If you've a special interest, pastime or hobby, why not develop it in company with other enthusiasts? Or if you haven't any particularly personal interest, why not start a new one?

If you are handicapped by blindness, deafness or some other disability, this need not bar you from club activities.

The Royal National Institute for the Blind	224 Great Portland Street London W1N 6AA Tel: 01–388 1266	9 Viewfield Place Stirling SK8 1NL Tel: 0786 3652
The Royal National Institute for the Deaf	105 Gower Street London WC1E 6AH Tel: 01–387 8033	9A Claremont Gardens Glasgow G3 7LW Tel: 041–332 0343
The Disabled Living Foundation	380/384 Harrow Road London W9 2HU Tel: 01–289 6111	Scottish Council on Disability Princes House 5 Shandwick Place Edinburgh EH2 4RS Tel: 031–229 8632

will all provide details of local clubs. You can also get information on local clubs and groups from a health visitor or social worker and from your local library or Citizens' Advice Bureau.

4 Get help with your worries

Anxiety can make you isolated. Don't keep your worries to yourself, share them with a local Citizens' Advice Bureau worker, or a social worker or with your doctor.

5 Tackle housing problems

Housing problems are often at the root of a person's loneliness. If you are unhappy in your housing situation, you may not want to invite people to your home, or there may be a physical problem, such as stairs, which keeps you housebound. Get help and advice on your worries in this field. If you are a council tenant, you can turn to your local housing management. Citizens' Advice Bureaux also give housing advice.

6 Take up a course of study
This is another guaranteed method of meeting people with similar interests. Adult Education classes cover a wide range of subjects at all levels of difficulty.

7 Get involved with your place of worship
This can mean joining a friendly and concerned community, sharing the same convictions. If transport is a problem, most congregations make a commitment to help less mobile members take part in services.

8 Invite a visitor
Why not invite a visitor into your home? Don't feel that you have nothing to give to other people because you're stuck at home — you can provide a refuge and a ready ear which your visitors will value.

9 Make a penfriend
There are a host of letter-writing clubs you can join, as well as keeping up correspondence with friends. Write enclosing a stamped addressed envelope to the International Friendship League (British Section)
Peacehaven
3 Creswick Road, Acton
London W3 9HE

10 Take a holiday
There are an increasing number of well organised group holidays which any single person can confidently look forward to enjoying. Disability need not exclude you — RADAR publish a list of holidays as do Age Concern.

Saga (Senior Citizens) Holidays Ltd
119 Sandgate Road
Folkestone
Kent CT20 2BN   Tel: 0303 47062

RADAR (Royal Association for Disability & Rehabilitation)
25 Mortimer Street
London W1N 8AB   Tel: 01–637 5400

Age Concern England
60 Pitcairn Road
Mitcham
Surrey CR4 3LL
Tel: 01–640 5431

Age Concern Scotland
33 Castle Street
Edinburgh
EH2 3DN
Tel: 031–225 5000

Living alone

One of the great assets of living with a partner is that someone else notices and cares about your moods and experiences. If you live on your own, it is not selfish to think about ways of providing support and kindness to yourself.

If you are feeling a bit depressed, or have just had an interesting encounter and are longing to talk about it, another person's concern and interest is almost essential. It is very easy to miss out on this kind of emotional support if you live alone.

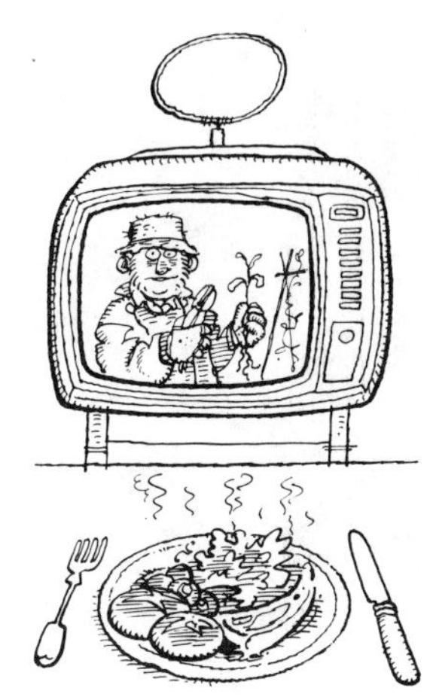

There is no reason why you should deny yourself the little daily pleasures of life, just because you're on your own. In fact, it's even more important to think about such things. A good meal, for instance, can be a real pleasure, but if you are low and depressed or lonely and can't be bothered to make an effort, you can fall into the habit of not preparing regular decent meals for yourself.

Watching your favourite television programme, or listening to the radio, is a very enjoyable activity. It can also provide a topic of conversation when you meet other people — especially if they like the same programme.

Sensual pleasures

Take a fresh look at what you eat, and where. A carefully laid table, attractive dishes and attention to presentation seem to make food taste better and improve your appetite. You don't need to be rich, or greedy, to derive pleasure from preparing and eating meals.

If you normally eat alone, why not suggest to a friend that you eat together? You can do this in a variety of ways — take turns to act as host, cook together or each contribute to a prepared part of the meal. This shouldn't cost you any more. The object is not to impress one another with your Cordon Bleu skills, rather to vary your routine by sharing a meal-time and perhaps stimulating one another to try something new, such as the unusual vegetables now being imported or a dish such as pizza, which may not have been part of your usual repertoire.

Looking after yourself

An idea which has made its way from the west coast of America into general use in recent years is that of **nurturing**, when applied to oneself. In the same way as a parent might provide enriching experiences, little treats, for a child, the idea is that you deliberately give yourself pleasant experiences, or try to be more aware of the ones which you already have in everyday life. It could be something very simple like drinking your morning cup of tea from a fine china cup or taking pleasure from the sight of a few wild flowers in a vase.

Which are the experiences or encounters which give you pleasure in your daily life? It is very easy, because of depression or the effect of routine, to fail to enjoy the ordinary pleasure of daily living.

As an experiment, try an 'awareness day'. Try to be very conscious of what you are doing; the clothes you wear, the food you eat, the people you talk to, books you read, radio or TV programmes, even the view from your window. Can you change your routine to build in little pleasures — eat your meal by the window instead of facing the kitchen wall perhaps? Your awareness day should help you to be more conscious of pleasure that need not be limited by disability or frailty.

Why not do something you may not have done for years, such as baking your own bread? Few of us are immune to the attractions of newly baked bread. The wholesome smell and the taste and texture feature in many people's memories of childhood. An added bonus is the satisfaction to be gained from making your own — making the 'staff of life' touches something deep in most of us, and it's good for arthritic joints too!

Touch

All of us, not just young babies, need human warmth and contact. Without it, we can fail to thrive. There is a good deal of truth in the cliche 'touch the body and you touch the heart'.

We all have areas of reserve about touching, although it seems to be the case that younger people are becoming less inhibited about this. For most of us, as we grow older, we touch one another less. In any school playground you will see little huddles of girls with their arms round one another, exchanging confidences; while their male contemporaries are more likely to be rolling on the ground, jumping on one another's backs or wrestling. But once childhood is past, most people become very selective about touching — a boy or girl friend, a spouse, one's children or other people's very young children — the list is usually fairly short.

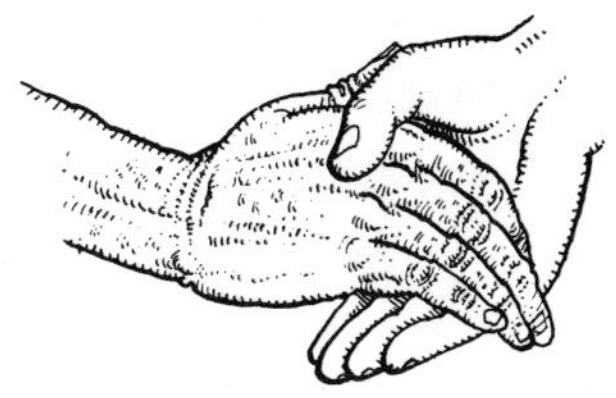

If you regret a lack of touching in your life, why not be brave and do something about it. Give a visitor a hug when she leaves or arrives or take her hand while she is talking to you. Because we don't touch one another much, as a rule, your visitor may be surprised, but usually delighted too. We gain pleasure from physical contact with other people, but are often too shy to make the first move.

Massage is very relaxing and pleasurable. Try massaging a friend's neck or shoulders, or get them to do it to you. There are many oils and creams available to make this more enjoyable.

You might like to think about people who have very little opportunity for human contact in their lives. Long stay patients in hospital, for example, may not have regular contact with relatives or friends.

Why not make a deliberate decision to befriend someone in this position, perhaps an older neighbour who is housebound or in residential care? Both of you can benefit enormously from this sort of friendship.

Loving and sex

Visitors from another planet, who based their opinion about love and sex in our society on what they saw in films, television and other media might assume that only young people were expected to have a sexual identity.

In the past, it has only been the most determined and self-confident older men and women who have been able to challenge the image of a sexless and often loveless old age.

What are the facts about older people and sexual capacity? Dr Alex Comfort, in his book, *A Good Age*, gives straightforward information which contradicts many of the usual myths.

"**Sex:** Ageing induces some changes in human sexual performance. These are chiefly in the male, for whom orgasm becomes less frequent. It occurs in every second act of intercourse, or in one act in three, rather than every time. More direct physical stimulation is also needed to produce an erection. However, compared with say, running ability, these changes are functionally minimal and actually tend in the direction of 'more miles per gallon' and greater, if less acute, satisfaction for both partners. In the absence of two disabilities — actual disease and the belief that 'the old' are or should be asexual — sexual requirement and sexual capacity are lifelong. Even if and when actual intercourse is impaired by infirmity, other sexual needs persist, including closeness, sensuality and being valued as a man or as a woman.

"The view is, of course, totally contrary to folklore . . . older people weren't asked in surveys about their sexual activity because everyone knew that they had none, and they were assumed to have none because nobody asked. Questions of this kind weren't asked by doctors either, because they might cause embarrassment, and they continued to cause embarrassment, although much less to the patient than to the doctor, because they weren't routinely asked."

The surveys of sexual behaviour which have been conducted in the past forty years all confirm the opinion Comfort expresses — that older men and women have always had active sexual lives — but have tended to keep quiet about it because younger people had such hostile attitudes to ageing sexuality.

Your sexuality is part of your personality. It can be expressed in a whole variety of ways, in the clothes that you choose, the perfume that you wear; there are no rules about what is right or wrong. How to express your sexuality is totally up to you.

Sexual potency

A situation where older men and women simply remained reticent about their sex lives in order not to upset the sensibilities of their children's generation might seem funny, or a bit sad, but it becomes more serious when older people need medical help and professional support.

Many older men experience problems of impotence or premature ejaculation and it is by no means certain that they will encounter the same support and advice offered by the medical profession as would be automatically available to a younger man.

One of the less publicised findings of a very large and well-known survey of American sexual behaviour done by Masters and Johnson was that any kind of therapy programme for impotence or premature ejaculation is equally applicable to all age groups, because most of these problems are psychological in origin and not physical. The researchers drew on their reports from older participants to suggest that ejaculation at every act of intercourse might be impossible for older men, but that they and their partners can adjust to this and to the need for rest periods of several days between orgasms. Even when an older man has a history of heart disease, there is no need to stop sexual activity unless heart disease is very severe. Most doctors now believe that the good it does outweighs the risks. It is important not to get over-tired and to find positions that avoid cramp and tension.

Problems are occasionally reported by men suffering from high blood pressure. It seems likely that the drugs used to control blood pressure are responsible for the impotence often associated with this condition. This is something to discuss with your doctor if you are being prescribed tablets for high blood pressure.

There seems to be abundant evidence that sexual capacity in women usually persists into old age. Though there may be physical changes in the extent and speed with which the vagina becomes lubricated, the pattern of arousal and orgasm remains the same. Dryness can cause discomfort, but there are many creams and lubricants which help to restore easy and pleasurable sexual contact.

However, while a woman's sexual capacity may remain the same, many older women no longer have the same opportunity for a regular sex life as they did in earlier years. There is evidence, however, that other reasons than a simple lack of a sexual partner may lead women to give up sexual activity long before their physical capacity is exhausted. Many older women are the victims of our society's hostile attitudes towards sexuality in later life.

Have you too been brainwashed a little? Think back to how you yourself felt about this issue twenty years ago, and compare your attitudes then to how you feel today:

> **1** Did you think that older couples should be satisfied with 'companionship' in marriage?
> **2** Did you find the idea that an older man or woman might be sexually active and satisfied somewhat disturbing?
> **3** Would you have been disturbed to learn that many older women take comfort in masturbation?

How do your attitudes now compare with what you thought twenty years ago — do you find that you have come to feel differently about these things as you have grown older?

There, but not there

There is a bitter loneliness that overtakes some men and women who are caring for a husband or wife who is suffering from brain-failure.

People with **Alzheimer's disease** or one of the other, less common forms of dementia have very often lost their memories of a shared life together and may show changes in personality which make them strangers to a husband or wife who has known them for many years.

The Alzheimer's Disease Society
Bank Buildings
Fulham Broadway
London SW16 1EP
01–381 3177

Alzheimer's Disease Society
40 Shandwick Place
Edinburgh EH2 4RT
031–225 1453

These organisations were set up to help the relatives of sufferers from this illness and they offer a telephone counselling service to carers who are at their wit's end trying to cope.

Do ask for help if this is your problem. Although in many areas there is a scandalously inadequate provision in the community, respite care may be available to some extent, through day hospitals, day care centres, sitting-in services etc.

A publication which offers practical guidance is *The 36-hour Day* by Nancy Mace and Peter Rabins. It is a family guide to caring for persons with Alzheimer's disease, related dementing illness and memory loss in later life. (John Hopkins University Press (1981), available from Winslow Press.)

Also, for enquiries from Scotland, there is *Coping with Dementia — A Handbook for Carers*, available from:

SHEG
Health Education Centre
Woodburn House
Canaan Lane
Edinburgh EH10 4SG

A partner who is doing a caring job needs to look after herself and you should look for all the outside support possible — the trouble is that someone who is coping with a situation near the limits of their capacity is not in a position to go looking for help, knocking on doors and waiting for appointments.

The Association of Carers
21-23 New Road
Chatham
Kent ME4 4QJ

is a self-help group of relatives who understand these pressures and who may be able to advise you. You can also get in touch with:

Crossroads Scotland Care Attendant Scheme
24 George Square
Glasgow G2 1EC

Looking to the future

Most women, when they married, chose or were chosen by a partner a little older than themselves. Women in western countries live, on average, slightly longer than men. These two factors give rise to some hard facts which concern all older women:

Most older persons are women.

Most older men are married.

Most married women are likely to outlive their husbands.

It is not morbid, but sensible, to look these facts in the eye **before** you are overtaken by them.

There are practical things you can do to prepare for this situation.

▶ You can both make your wills. This need not be expensive. A standard will form is legal provided it is witnessed by someone who will not profit from the will, or you may prefer to consult a solicitor.

▶ If you have a family car, can you drive it? Do you have any idea what it costs to run — including insurance?

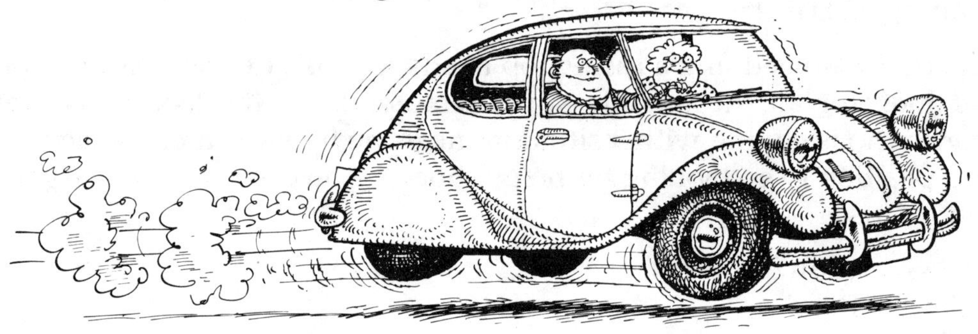

▶ Do you know what your financial position would be if your husband died?

▶ What about your housing? If you have paid off a mortgage on your own home, is there money for essential repairs?

▶ Do you know what needs to be done **immediately** when someone dies? There is an excellent Consumer Association guide *What to do when someone dies*. It might be a good idea to get a copy now, when you don't need it, to save adding bewilderment about officialdom to the grief of a loss.

▶ Have you and your spouse talked about what you would like done? If one of you has strong feelings about, for instance, cremation or leaving your eyes for corneal grafting, have you discussed this?

Two organisations which may like to contact for help in beginning again after a bereavement are:

Cruse
126 Sheen Road
Richmond
Surrey
Tel: 01–940 4818

Cruse
3 Rutland Square
Edinburgh
EH1 2AS
Tel: 031–229 6275

National Association of Widows
Stafford and District Voluntary Services
Chell Road
Stafford
Tel: 0785 45465

None of us, as we grow older, escape the experience of loss and bereavement. To the loss of loved relatives and friends there may be added loss of mobility, loss of strength and capacity, loss of an accustomed home and occupation.

There are no easy answers to offer to people adjusting to loss in their lives, but we can allow people to share their experiences and not allow our own shyness to discourage friends from talking about their grief.

Grieving has bad effects on both physical and mental health. Bereavement, in common with other major life changes, can make people ill. For instance, one study which compared GPs' case-notes on a group of widows in the eighteen months following bereavement with the records on the same women in the previous eighteen months showed a marked increase in consultations with their doctors. Most of these women asked for sedatives or 'tonics' to help with the physical side-effects of grief.

A similar study of admissions to a psychiatric hospital showed that admission for an illness which arose after the death of a marriage partner occurred seven times more frequently than would normally have been expected.

Grieving can thus have effects on both physical and mental health. Is there any way these bad effects can be avoided?

If you have lost a loved husband or wife, there may be some comfort in the knowledge that some of the strange things you do are quite common and a part of the bereaved person's struggle to really 'take in' what has happened to them. An extra torment that many bereaved people suffer is the fear that they may be going mad — perhaps they talk to a dead husband or wife, lay a place at the table for him, hear her footsteps in the hall or may see the dead person sitting in a favourite chair or standing by a window. Many people speak of an awareness of the lost person's 'presence' and of the comfort that this brings — it hardly seems important whether this is conjured up by grief or is objectively real. Talking about her own experience, Mrs Hargraves told us:

"For a while I'd just get up in the morning and set the table for breakfast after they'd gone to work and very often I'd find myself putting his cup and saucer . . . and I suddenly realised . . . It took me two years really to get over it, I don't think I would have done, but with the help of the children and the family."

It can help to know what to expect and to realise that what you are going through is a common experience. Colin Murray Parkes, a psychiatrist who has made special studies of grief, describes four stages of normal grieving.

1 **Numbness and disbelief.** This is the most frequent immediate response to a death and can last from a few hours to several days.

2 **Yearning and protest.** The bereaved person is tense and hyper-active, suffering severe pangs of grief and painful pining. The individual is completely preoccupied with the lost person and will go over the events surrounding the death repeatedly. Resentment is often felt against doctors, relatives, friends, or against God.

3 **Depression and disorganisation.** A sense of aimlessness and lack of purpose are characteristic of this stage, but it should not last for more than 3 months if it is to pass on to:

4 **Reorganisation.** This stage occurs when depression gradually subsides and there is a re-awakening of interest in normal activities. This stage is

is often associated with having got past the first anniversary of the death.

Sometimes people do not pass through the four stages of grief and instead experience chronic grief, in which the individual is still suffering acute anguish two or three years after bereavement. This is particularly likely to happen when there has been a **very dependent relationship**, in which loss of a husband means also loss of a job, social contacts, a whole identity, together with elaborate plans for a future which will not now come about.

It is important to look at your relationship with your spouse while you are both still fit and well and to face up to the question of how one of you, left alone, will cope.

Grieving can also persist beyond the usual when there is:

Lack of opportunity to grieve. A person may, after a death, involve him or herself in physical work and perhaps deliberately not find time to express their feelings. The person may also have strong ideas about not showing emotion or breaking down and will preserve a rigid front of reserve. It seems evident that postponed or inhibited grief is likely to lead to long-term difficulties and that the expression of grief is somehow necessary for us all if we are to come through acute grieving to a more tranquil state of mind.

Our own deaths

For some of us, the loss which preoccupies our thoughts is of our own death, rather than the loss of loved friends and relatives.

One of the ideas which is commonly voiced about older people is that 'they' are preoccupied with death and full of fears about their own dying. However, the research that has been done on this subject, most of it conducted in America, suggests that this is not true. In one study, interviewers asked several thousand people to respond to this question:

"Some people say that they are afraid to die, and others say that they are not. How do you feel?"

The answers were grouped into five categories:

▶ terrified;

▶ afraid;

▶ neither afraid nor unafraid;

▶ unafraid;

▶ eager.

Few people of any age said that they were terrified of death and it was those in the youngest age group (20–39) who most frequently said that they were afraid, and were the least likely to say that they were unafraid or eager. The researchers found much less fear of death among the old than among the young.

Many older people do, however, express a fear of painful or protracted dying, or of continuing to live on in a helpless state.

"For many years I had the care of my mother whose warm, loving, active life was gradually extinguished by the demands of a body which made her totally dependent upon others. By the time she was in her nineties, keeping her alive involved a daily struggle for both of us. Should I ever suffer the same disabilities, involving the constant attention of other people, I would not wish to live. Human dignity is not compatible with such a condition, when the dignity and meaning of life has vanished."

Mrs Elizabeth Merson

Do you share Mrs Merson's attitude? Have you ever talked about this issue with those close to you? In a postscript to her letter to us Mrs Merson added:

"In all the long years during which my mother and I lived together she never at any time mentioned the word **death**! I believe her deep fear of dying was increased by her inability to discuss the subject."

This insight about her mother is amply confirmed by the work of the psychiatrist Elisabeth Kubler-Ross. She worked with groups of terminally ill patients in Chicago and found that the opportunity to talk was the greatest benefit that could be offered to men and women struggling to come to terms with their own deaths. Far from being depressing reading her book offers support and comfort. You may like to try and obtain it; the title is *On Death and Dying* and it was published in 1973 by Tavistock Publications.

Reaching out

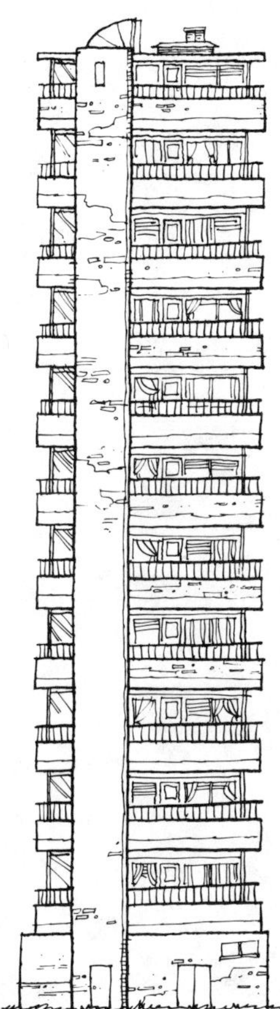

It's all very well encouraging a lonely person to 'get out of doors and meet people'. But to a really lonely person like Mrs Fairfield, a widow who gave up her job and social life to nurse her husband, going out only emphasises her isolation:

"I get tidied up and walk all the way up the town to the big Safeway. I go all round the shop and get a loaf, which is all I really need, and then go and have a cup of tea in the cafe upstairs. I don't see a soul I know and don't speak to anyone. By the time I've trailed all the way home again and gone up in the lift to my flat on the twelfth floor, I feel ready to jump out of the window."

Given the British passion for 'keeping ourselves to ourselves', friendships or even casual social contacts are not going to develop without a little help. One way to develop friendships is through a shared interest, and learning a new skill is itself satisfying, whether or not it leads to new friends.

Do consider learning something totally new to you. An adult education class is not the first thing most older people think of when they are looking for company and occupation. Only a small percentage of Britain's 10 million older people enrol in classes; perhaps because of anxieties about expense, worries about being out of the house late in the evening, a feeling that it is only for more 'educated' people or an impression that education is only for the young. But learning in later life is for everyone.

Taking up opportunities to learn in later life can give a tremendous boost to self-confidence. One of the greatest advocates of continuing education for older people was Gladys Elder. In her book *The Alienated*, on growing old today, she describes how the chance of education offered her an escape route from the dehumanising effects of retirement, bereavement and increasing deafness. She began with a correspondence course and later went on to take an Open University degree course.

"I came to terms for the first time with my failing senses and decided it would not be the end whatever happened, as long as I kept my mental and critical faculties alive . . . I have learned more in the past few years than in many previous years and thus my life has been enriched."

(Gladys Elder OAP, *The Alienated: Growing Old Today*. Published by the Writers and Readers Publishing Co-operative 1977.)

But learning something new need not be a very serious business. Drop in to your local leisure centre or Adult Education Institute. A great variety of courses are available, both day and evening, from cookery and car maintenance to yoga and wine-making. Many Institutes offer special introductory 'taster' days for older people, where you can go along and try something without committing yourself to enrolling for a full course. You can almost certainly find day-time classes, if you are worried about going out in the evening.

Nowadays, local schools are much more orientated towards links with the community than they used to be. Older people, young mothers and others at home during the day are often encouraged to take an active part in the daily life of their local school.

Miss Ada Thompson is a widow in her eighties living in Gateshead. She was invited to take part in a project called **Side by Side** in which older people worked alongside children in the classroom on a variety of craft and history projects.

"I taught them how to make 'stotty cake'. It's an old Tyneside recipe for flat loaves. The women used to make them last thing on a baking day and they cooked as the oven cooled down. The children had never heard of it — their Mums don't bake like we did — and they were so interested. We had them making proggy mats out of old rags cut up in strips too. That's another old craft that's gone now."

In this scheme old and young found they had a great deal to offer one another. Do ask at your local school if there is any way you might become involved in such a project. You could also write to Help the Aged, who encourage schools and youth groups to set up projects involving older people. Write to:

Education & Research Department
Help the Aged
Education
FREEPOST
London EC1B 1BD

Planning to get away for a short break is a tremendous boost to your morale. Why not combine a holiday break with trying out something new and a bit challenging?

One way to try out a new experience is to take a weekend course or short break at a field centre or with a tour operator specialising in learning and activity holidays.

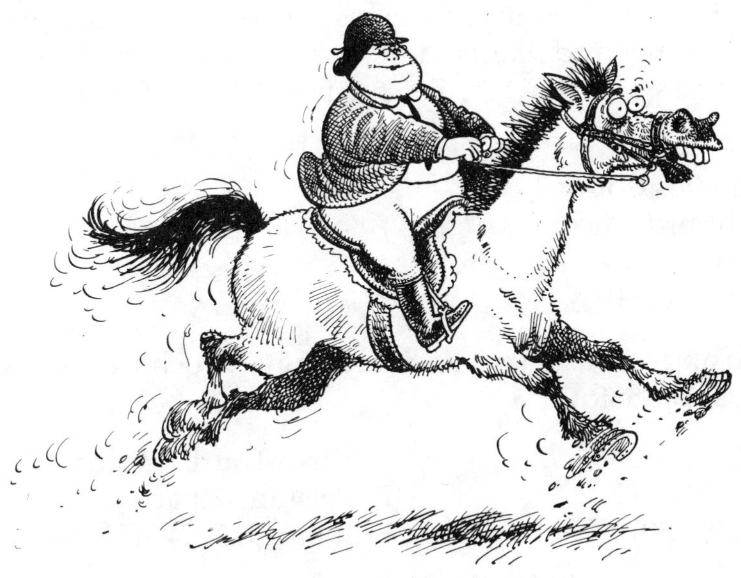

You can even try your hand at vigorous activities such as canoeing, pony-trekking and sailing. The YMCA have recently started a programme of adventure holidays for older people in the Lake District, co-ordinated by trained instructors.

Write to:

YMCA National Centre
Lakeside
Ulverston
Cumbria LA12 8BD

The Peak National Park has a residential study centre for field studies and fell walkers in the Peak District. They also have a special programme called Exploring the Peak District for the Over-50s. Write to:

Losehill Study Centre
Castleton
Derbyshire S30 2WB

The Field Studies Council has a wide range of short courses at field centres throughout the country. Courses range from painting and drawing to photography and crafts and various aspects of ecology and conservation, birds and flowers. For further details of their programmes write to:

The Field Studies Council
Preston Montford
Montford Bridge
Shrewsbury SY4 1HW

The Scottish and English Tourist Boards have brochures of activity and hobby holidays. Write to:

Admail 14
London SW1W 0YC
(and enclose £1.50)

Scottish Tourist Board
Ravelston Terrace
Edinburgh EH4 3EF

You may also find copies in your local library.

If you are managing a disability and are wholly or partly housebound, opportunities to pursue activities and interests that take you out of the house are even more important. Two older women who would otherwise have been house-bound described the help they received:

"I have just come back from Mundesley Holiday Camp with a Social Worker and had a wonderful time as she took me in all the shops. I haven't been in a shop since I went to Wood Green with the disabled last December."
Nellie Linsell
"Kind friends collect us for visits to their homes occasionally, and I have discovered that my water colour paintings are pleasing enough to be accepted. I find this stimulating."
D D Copsey
Many organisations exist to help people with disabilities to have a break from home. RADAR publish a range of books and literature on aids, ideas and facilities for disabled people. This includes *Holidays for the Physically Handicapped*. Please write to:

RADAR (Royal Association for Disability and Rehabilitation)
25 Mortimer Street
London W1N 8AB

Scottish Council on Disability
Princes House
5 Shandwick Place
Edinburgh EH2 4RG

Another useful guide is *Holidays for the Handicapped* published by the Automobile Association.

GRACE (Mrs Gould's Residential Advisory Service for the Elderly) may be able to help you if you are looking for hotels or guest houses who can also provide extra help or nursing support if you or a partner require it. Write to:

GRACE
PO Box 71
Cobham, Surrey KT11 2JR

Arthritis Care also have a number of holiday centres and self-catering units specifically adapted to meet the needs of arthritis sufferers.

For further information write to:

Arthritis Care
6 Grosvenor Crescent
London SW1X 7ER

Even the most contented and self-sufficient of us occasionally feels lonely — it's possible to feel very lonely in the midst of a loving family, or with a partner or in a big crowd. This section has been about making plans to tackle feelings of isolation, developing occupations and interests and involving ourselves with other people. Two older people who have made the effort to join groups and evening classes described what it meant to them.

Mrs Green, who is a widow living by herself in a flat in the centre of Newcastle has become a regular visitor to a Drop-in centre:

"I've got all the pains in the world when I'm at home . . . when I go swimming and dancing and keep fit I forget all about them."

Miss Hodgson goes regularly to two evening classes:

"When I get home sometimes, with housework to do, I think, 'why am I doing this?' I'm putting all this energy in and wonder why. But if I sit down and think about it, I'm doing it because it gives me extra happiness."

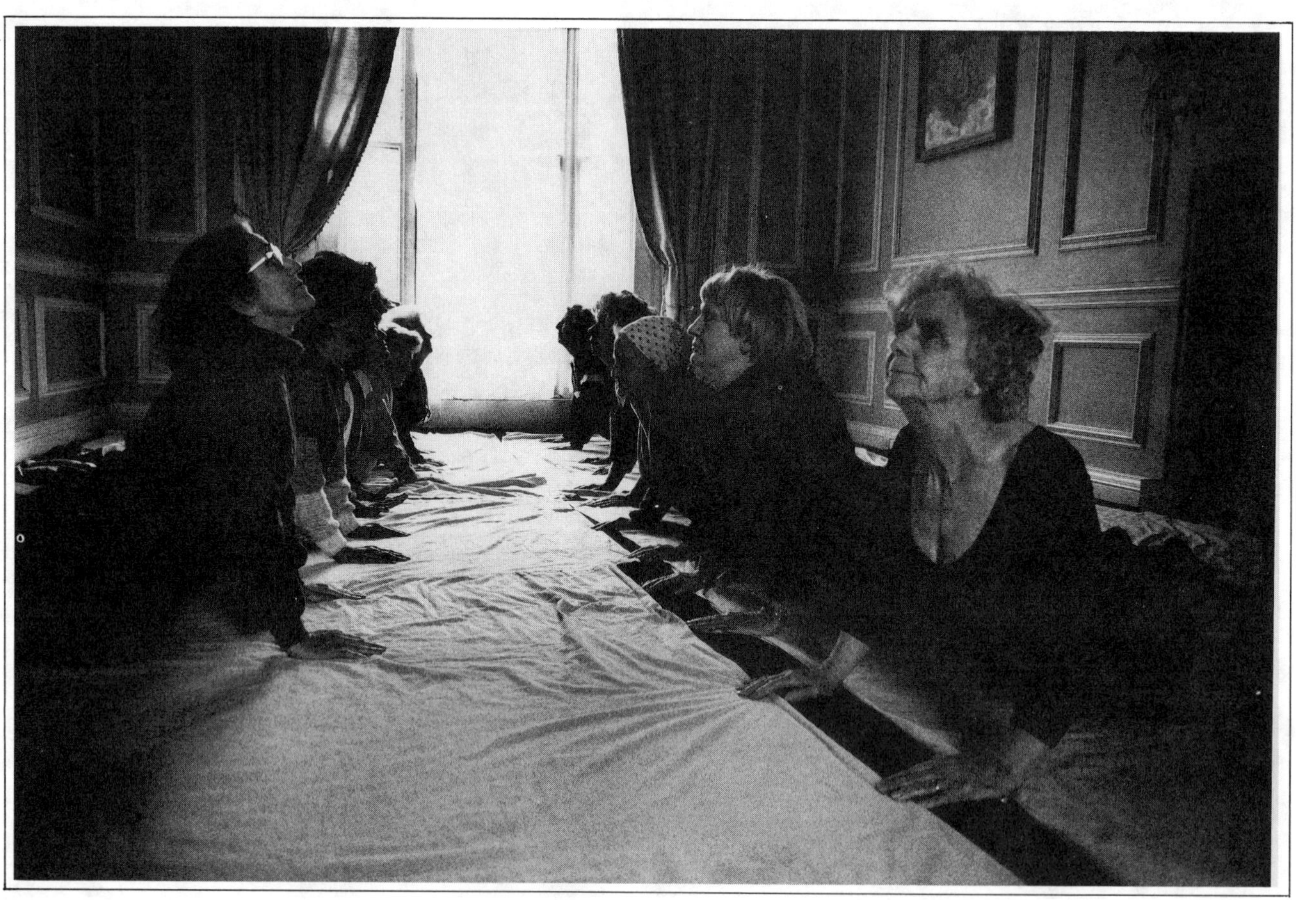

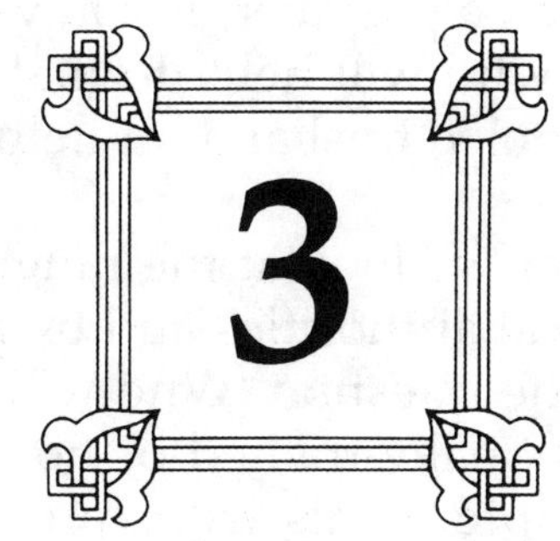

3

YOU AND THE SYSTEM: WHO HELPS?

If you are ill and need help, you probably turn to your GP, or to a member of the family, who will contact your doctor on your behalf. But sometimes the situation is not so cut and dried. You may feel that you need help, but don't know who to turn to for advice and assistance. If your drain is blocked you need a plumber, if you've broken your leg you need hospital treatment, but who will help if what you need is a break from full-time care of your disabled husband, or help with your shopping or to visit your dentist?

In this chapter we look at the range of services which are provided by the state, by local authorities and by private and voluntary agencies. We try to answer the question 'Who will help?' and we look at the range of people, professionally trained or not, who give personal care. Although most of the chapter deals with care provided by the health service, we consider that many other factors, such as housing, transport and community services can also affect health. We are considering health in the widest possible sense, and will look at the work of people such as social workers, home helps, day centre staff, voluntary workers and good neighbours in supporting older people in their own homes.

The National Health Service

The NHS began in 1948, with the aim of giving everyone access to the medical care they needed, whether or not they could afford to pay for it. It is funded mainly from central government funds, raised by taxation, with only a small contribution to the real cost being made by National Insurance contributions and charges to patients for prescriptions etc.

Health care available under the NHS is either available in the community or is provided in hospital.

Community services include all those services to which a member of the general public has open access, eg. you can visit your doctor or dentist merely by phoning to make an appointment. Health workers in the Community Services are often described as belonging to a **primary health care team** and include GPs, health visitors and community nurses; sometimes social workers, dentists, opticians and pharmacists are included in the team. The general practitioner is the linchpin of the primary health care team and you gain access to it by registering with a doctor. In England GPs within the health service are under contract with their **Family Practitioner Committee** and are listed in a register which is held by the committee and by the local Community Health Council. In Scotland the situation is slightly different and GPs work under contract to the Primary Health Care Division of the Health Board.

Specialist and hospital services include, as well as Accident and Emergency Departments, all the secondary services under the NHS. In order to gain access to these, you must be referred by a GP to a hospital consultant. You will either be seen as an out-patient, examined in your own home or admitted to hospital according to the nature of your complaint.

A general practitioner is obliged to refer a patient to a specialist working within the NHS if this is necessary, but no doctor need refer you to a specialist just because you want to see one. If you are determined to see a consultant despite your doctor's opinion, you will have to change your doctor, or else visit a GP in private practice and ask for a private referral.

Let's look at the people you will meet when you come into the sphere of the professional health worker, at what they do and how they react to the rest of us.

Most of us meet professionals within the health service at moments when we ourselves are at a low ebb. If you're scared and in pain, and they've written out an exhaustive family history, stuck needles in you and taken blood samples, asked you to provide a urine sample, given you unpleasant things to swallow, pinned up charts which concern you but are hung where you can't read them and — final indignity — taken away your outdoor clothes, you're not likely to be feeling your normal, assertive and competent self. On the contrary, faced with this situation, most of us go back to a childhood state of mind in which we want the clever, grown-up doctors and nurses to look after us and tell us what to do.

This is obviously not true for everyone. The stress of being ill may cause some individuals to fight back vigorously, to try to assert themselves in a situation where they feel at a disadvantage.

Professional health workers are trained to be aware of the stress involved in being ill. They are also aware that patients don't just need to be told that everything is going to be all right. Many of us would like to achieve a situation in which we collaborate with the professionals in maintaining our good health and planning strategies for our future health care.

You and your doctor

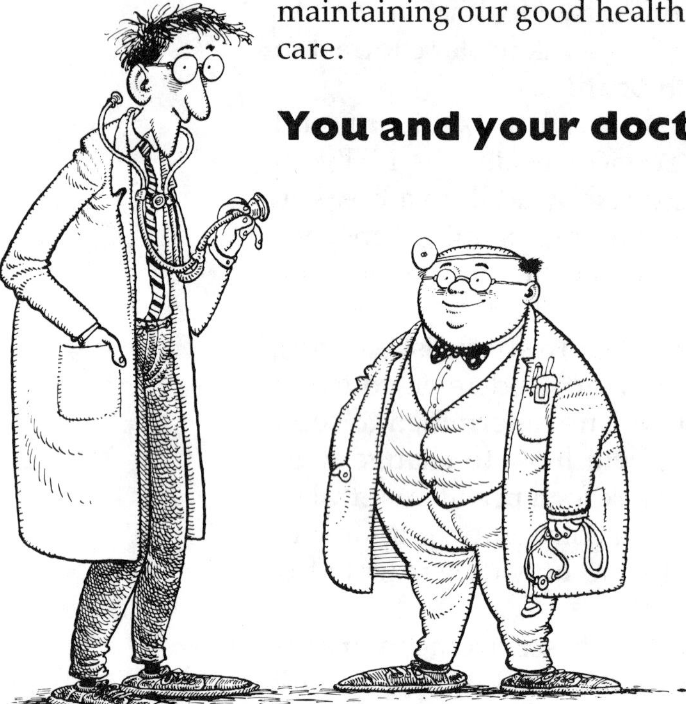

Like patients, doctors come in all shapes and sizes and with styles that range from the old-fashioned 'bedside manner' to those committed to 'patient participation'. Despite individual attitudes there are, however, certain services which all doctors provide for their patients. You can visit your doctor by appointment or be visited in your home if you are unable to make the trip to the surgery. Doctors are bound to make arrangements for a twenty-four hour service, either by sharing a rota with other GPs in their practice or by employing a deputising service. The whole question of access to a GP and what happens when a doctor is not available can be a source of friction and complaint. Doctors are understandably irritated by being asked to make a home visit to a patient who could easily visit the surgery, while patients complain of receptionists who block their access to the doctor, of group practices in which they never see the same doctor twice, or of problems in contacting deputising services in an emergency. Typical of patients' complaints is this comment from one older lady:

"What I feel is rather annoying and frustrating is the appointment system. It seems that you have to know in advance when you will be ill. Unless it is desperately urgent, you can never get an appointment on the day you need to see a doctor, or even on the following day. By the time you get one you are usually much better or much worse!"

If you are generally dissatisfied with the arrangements to see your doctor, in and outside surgery hours, do let your doctor know how you feel. Difficulties can often be resolved by speaking out and finding out the real facts of the situation.

If, however, you decide that no progress can be made and that you would prefer to change your doctor, you may find it hard to get a place on the list of another doctor in the same area. You should first seek an interview with the doctor of your choice, who is likely to ask you why you wish to change.

A doctor is unlikely to accept a patient who is assumed to be 'difficult', so it may be tactful to confine your comments to a simple statement that you have failed to develop a good relationship with your present GP. Your new doctor will fill in Part A on your medical card which you should then take or send to your old doctor. You do not need to give your reasons for wishing to make a change. The Health Service is obliged to find a doctor for patients who cannot do so on their own. In England this is the responsibility of the Family Practitioner Committees and, in Scotland, of your local Health Board.

Helping your GP to help you

Many people have had the experience of emerging from a consultation with their doctor feeling frustrated and confused. Particularly if you have vivid memories of pre-NHS days, you may be very anxious not to 'bother the doctor' with all your troubles, or shyness may mean that you don't get round to explaining what is **really** worrying you until the end of the interview. Occasionally, people may have another reason for not telling the doctor what is worrying them. As one older lady said frankly:

"I don't want him to tell me anything I don't want to hear."

It is **always** better to speak out about something which is worrying you, rather than hugging it to yourself as a secret. Very often a simple remedy is available and, even when your fears of a serious disease are justified, prompt attention can greatly improve your chances of recovery. Although your doctor can learn a great deal from examining you, you will need to tell him or her what is worrying you, if you are to be properly advised. Some well-tried ideas for making sure you get the help you need:

> ▶ Write down beforehand the symptoms you want to mention, or points you want to raise with your doctor.
> ▶ Don't hesitate to ask if you don't understand anything that is said.
> ▶ Do take a friend or relative along with you, if you think you may not remember everything that is said or would feel more confident if someone else was there.
> ▶ Say what is worrying you most, first, instead of leaving it till you are nearly ready to leave.
> ▶ Describe your symptoms accurately and leave the diagnosis to the professional.
> ▶ Do **listen** as well as talk to your doctor during a consultation.

Older people who spoke to us about their doctors are, on the whole, very happy with the attention they receive from them. Many older people have memories of health care before the Second World War and of family worries about being able to pay the doctor's bill. The experience has ensured that they are among the staunchest defenders of the National Health Service and speak highly of the care they have received from GPs working within it.

"I've a lady doctor who's looked after me extremely well, and I couldn't wish for better treatment."

"My doctor's wonderful, absolutely wonderful."

Is this sort of high opinion always justified? Doctors are unlikely to make the mistake of lumping all 'old people' together as is too often done by the general public. They have too much experience of the wide range of health conditions among older people, from the fit and active to the very frail and dependent. And it is unusual today to meet a doctor who tells you 'It's your age'. However, doctors may occasionally make older people feel that their illnesses are boring and beyond help. Older people spoke to us about their feeling that they were not considered of equal importance:

"Some doctors today haven't got any patience with older people and they leave them longer than they should do."

And speaking of the doctor of a friend,

"Over the months he leaves it longer and longer between visits and he mostly comes at lunch-time and he'll have more to say to her daughter in the kitchen than he does to her."

Professional care and attention is not enough; we should also be able to come away from a GP's surgery feeling that we have been listened to and had our views respected.

Community nurses

This title is given to nurses who work outside hospitals in the community. They may have different training and jobs.

A **practice nurse** or **attached nurse** is a qualified nurse who works in a doctor's surgery.

You can often go directly to the practice nurse for treatment, such as a wound to be stitched or dressed or for a procedure such as having your ears syringed to remove accumulated wax. Practice nurses have the opportunity to build up long-term relationships with patients and can be a source of advice and help. They can advise you on diet, for instance, or on managing a chronic complaint such as arthritis. **A health visitor** is a qualified nurse who has taken an extra additional year of training, which concentrates on prevention of ill health and health education. You can approach a health visitor directly, without a referral from your GP — simply phone the surgery and ask to speak to her or have her contact you at a convenient time.

The greater part of a health visitor's work is done with young mothers and their babies, but they also have a responsibility towards the older people in their area.

She has an advisory, supporting role and can tell you what services are supplied locally by the NHS, the local authority and voluntary organisations. Her training has equipped the health visitor to help you to live as independently as possible. Health visitors have also had experience in counselling and are used to offering support in times of crisis such as the loss of a loved partner.

Outside the profession the range of knowledge and skills of health visitors is not always appreciated and they are seen as just 'nurses'. Your health visitor ought to be someone who has time to talk to you, is free to visit your home and will be able to offer constructive help — for instance, by applying on your behalf for an aid or adaptation to your home such as a handrail or bathing aid.

A **district nurse** or **community nurse** is a registered nurse who has taken a special course in home nursing. District nurses are often assisted by auxiliaries, who are practical nurses working under supervision. They carry out simple caring tasks such as bathing and changing dressings. District nurses work much more with older patients than do health visitors. They are in a position to recognise problems as they arise and to ensure that patients receive prompt and appropriate treatment.

Pharmacists

You may have noticed an advertising campaign in the magazines urging people to make good use of the professional help available from local pharmacists.

Like GPs, pharmacists are under contract to their local Family Practitioner Committees in England, and to the Health Boards in Scotland. These authorities keep lists of all those working within their area. The list gives the addresses and opening hours of all the prescribing chemists in the district. There is a standard charge for every item prescribed by a doctor, but large groups of the population are exempt from these.

Men and women over the statutory retirement age are exempt. You should also be exempt if you are a War Service pensioner requiring prescriptions for the disablement which qualifies you for the pension.

If you have not yet reached retirement age and are not eligible for exemption on grounds of low income, you may be interested in buying

pre-payment certificates for prescriptions. You pay in advance for a certificate lasting either four or twelve months and receive free prescriptions for that period. You will benefit if you need more than five items in four months or fifteen during the year. There is no refund available if you find you do not need all these items, and you may end up paying more than the prescriptions would have cost.

A pharmacist is not a doctor and if you are seriously worried about your health, you should consult your GP. However, you may want some advice on a problem which appears too trivial to take to the doctor. Ask to speak to the pharmacist, rather than just asking whoever is behind the counter, and be as clear as possible about your symptoms. The pharmacist will advise you to visit your doctor, if the illness seems at all serious or has lasted more than a few days.

Many people report problems with the so-called 'child-proof' packaging of modern drugs. If you have difficulty with fiddly packaging, you can ask for your pills to be supplied in an ordinary screw-topped bottle.

If you have a complaint against a pharmacist it should be made to the pharmacist's employer, who is either the Health Board Primary Care Division (in Scotland) or the Family Practitioner Committee.

Dentists

Not all dentists undertake NHS work. Check this when you make an appointment. Although many people visit the same dentist year after year, you do not need to register with a dentist and could, if you wanted, try a different one for each course of treatment you require.

Once you have chosen your dentist, you will be asked to sign a form which is, in effect, a contract between you and the dentist for a particular course of treatment. Make it clear at this stage that you wish to be treated on the NHS. If you cannot find a dentist who will accept you as an NHS patient, you can get advice from the employing authority, which is either the Family Practitioner Committee or the Health Board (in Scotland). You may wish to go privately or have treatment under the NHS at a dental hospital.

How much will I have to pay?

Except for young people, pregnant women and those on a low income, there is a charge for most NHS treatment. Some dentists may refuse to do complicated work such as bridges, dentures or crowns under the NHS. For some types of complex and expensive work, the dentist has to obtain approval from the **Dental Estimates Board** before he can provide treatment under the NHS. The board does refuse some applications, usually suggesting a cheaper treatment, but you may appeal against its decisions if you wish — to a hearing held by the DHSS.

You will not have to pay for dental treatment if you receive a Supplementary Pension* or Housing Benefit Supplement. You will also qualify for free treatment if, after deducting the cost of life insurance premiums, hire purchase payments for essential furniture and household equipment, and fares to hospital, your income is not more than £2.50 above the Supplementary Pension level. (As at 1987.)

Even if you are not eligible for free treatment, you may only have to pay reduced charges. The maximum that you can be charged is three times the amount by which your net income exceeds the qualifying level for free treatment (the Supplementary Pension level plus £2.50). So if your net income was £2.50 more than the qualifying level the most you would have to pay would be £7.50. You should also note that charges which occur within three weeks of each other will be lumped together and treated as one charge.

If you do not qualify for free dental treatment or reduced charges, the maximum you can be asked to pay for a course of treatment under the NHS is £115 (1987).

Some dentists provide emergency cover outside surgery hours, but they do not have to do this. In an emergency you can go to a hospital Accident and Emergency Department, where they will stop bleeding or give relief for severe pain.

A dentist who sees a patient in an emergency is not obliged to complete a course of treatment and make the patient 'dentally fit'.

---

* after April 1988 this extra help will be described differently.

The hospital dental service provides specialist treatment and major treatment such as the extraction of wisdom teeth.

If you are in hospital and cannot see your usual dentist, the hospital service will provide dental treatment. This is free, except for the supply of dentures and other appliances.

We asked older people to tell us about their experience of the dental service. Amongst reports of good care we received a good deal of complaint. Some was due to lack of knowledge about, for instance, charges, so that people were afraid to ask for treatment through fear of high costs. We were also told about the problems people had encountered in having dentures repaired and in locating dentists willing to do NHS work. Problems of access to surgeries were also reported, particularly in the cities where dentists often have premises upstairs.

Perhaps one reason for the poor communication between elderly people and their dentists is the change that has taken place in dentistry itself in recent years. Emphasis today is much more on saving people's own teeth if at all possible and it is much less common to 'have 'em all out and be done with it'. Denture wearers do seem to have difficulty finding sympathetic care, under the NHS.

Simplifying the system and making information about costs easily available would go a long way towards dealing with most of the main anxieties people have about dental treatment. See leaflet DS 11, available from the Post Office.

Chiropodists

In most areas there are too few chiropodists in the NHS.

Chiropody treatment under the NHS is available for men and women of pensionable age, schoolchildren, handicapped people and pregnant women. Chiropodists work in health centres, welfare clinics, old-people's homes, purpose-built clinics and hospitals. If you are house-bound you can be visited by a chiropodist, or you may be able to get transport provided by social services (in England), the Social Work Department (Scotland) or the ambulance service.

There is nothing to prevent anyone who wishes to do so from sticking a plaque on his front door advertising his services as a chiropodist.

Unqualified practitioners are notorious for the harm done to their victims' feet, for example by using corrosive chemicals to treat verrucas and corns. State-registered chiropodists will have spent three years training and they are the only chiropodists eligible to work within the NHS. If you pick a chiropodist from the yellow pages, you should look for the letters SRCh after the name, which establish that the individual is a state registered chiropodist. Members or fellows of the Society of Chiropodists will also have the initials MChS or FChS.

Because of the demand for NHS treatment and the shortage of qualified chiropodists there is no guarantee that you will be treated promptly. You can write to the District Chiropodist or to the Unit Administrator of the Health Board (Scotland) or District Health Authority (England) if you think you are experiencing an unreasonable delay in treatment.

However, many people do give up waiting and go privately. The Society of Chiropodists estimates that less than half of its members work full-time in the NHS. In some places, because of the shortage of NHS care, your GP may be able to refer you to a private chiropodist, whose fees will be met by the NHS.

Opticians

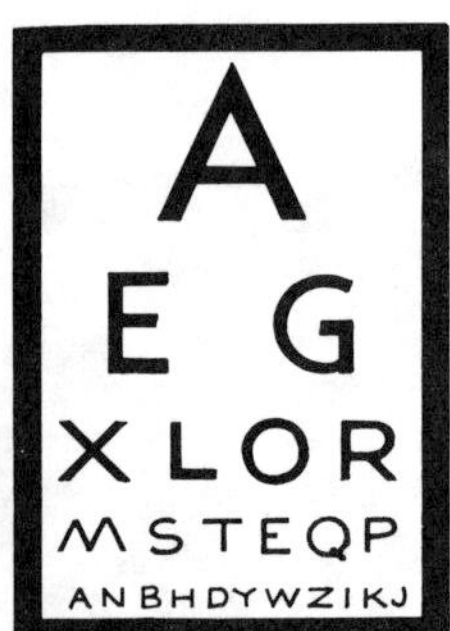

Opticians work under contract to the National Health Service. You do not need a referral to see an ophthalmic or dispensing optician, or to visit an ophthalmic medical practitioner (who usually works in a medical eye centre) but you do need to be referred by your GP to see a consultant ophthalmologist (eye specialist).

Most eye tests are done by ophthalmic opticians, or you may choose to visit a medical eye centre. If you are house-bound, a local optician may have a home-visiting service or you could have a home eye test provided by the Hospital Eye Service, on request from your GP. Alternatively, your health visitor may be able to arrange transport for you.

If you do need glasses the optician will give you a prescription which will be valid for two years.

Glasses are no longer available directly from the NHS but you may still qualify for help in the form of vouchers. You will qualify for a voucher if you are receiving a Supplementary Pension or Housing Benefit Supplement. If you do not receive Supplementary Benefit but still have a low income then you should get form F1 from your optician, fill it in, and send it to the DHSS. They in turn will send you form F3 (0) telling you if you qualify for help and if so how much. You will also qualify for help if you need complex/powerful lenses.

The advantage of this system is that you can shop around for glasses. But you should bear in mind that one recent survey found that prices can vary enormously for spectacles of the same quality.

The Hospital Service

"I found the doctors and nurses very kind."
"I found the doctors very friendly and helpful."
"They worked so hard, they were so kind."
"The doctors and nurses were all very kind."
"I've had marvellous treatment from doctors in hospital."

These are only snippets from the many letters which we received from older men and women who had been in hospital. There are the odd moans, often directed against domestic staff or porters rather than medical staff, but the general tone of our correspondence about the hospital service was, as we might have expected, one of grateful appreciation.

If you do have to come into hospital, who will you meet and what are their jobs?

Out-Patients Consultation

Once referred for an out-patient consultation, the speed with which you receive an appointment will depend on how serious your condition is and whereabouts in the country you live.

The **Consultants** do not personally see every patient referred to them.

Some patients will be seen by the registrar or house officer. Consultants work in a team which consists of

> Consultant
> Senior Registrar
> Registrar
> Senior House Officer
> House Officer

Smaller hospitals may not have all these staff in the team.

You cannot insist on seeing the consultant personally but you need not worry about getting 'inferior' treatment from a registrar or house officer.

The doctor will explain what is wrong with you and what further treatment is recommended. You need not feel too anxious if you don't understand everything that is said. Sometimes, if you are feeling nervous, you may not 'take in' what you are told; but your GP will receive a letter after your first consultation which you can ask about and so clarify anything that is worrying you.

Help with costs of visiting hospital

You may be able to claim for fares to hospital, either as an out-patient or as an in-patient. You will qualify for help if you receive Supplementary Pension or if your income would be less than Supplementary Pension levels after paying fares.

If you are an in-patient you should fill in form H11 at least seven days before being discharged. If you receive a Supplementary Pension your claim will be approved automatically. If not, you or your family will be visited to see if you are eligible.

Out-patients who receive a Supplementary Pension and have an order book should show this to the hospital receptionist or social worker who will arrange payment. If you do not have an order book ask the DHSS or hospital for form H11. The same applies if you do not receive a Supplementary Pension but think you may be eligible for help.

If you need the money for fares beforehand, rather than claiming it afterwards, you should explain this, either to the hospital or to the DHSS.

The money will then be made available.

You will get the fare for the cheapest form of public transport to the hospital. If there is no public transport then you should get a taxi to the nearest point at which it is available. The fares of an escort will also be paid if the hospital say that it is necessary.

Admission

If the consultant decides that you need in-patient treatment you will, unless it is an emergency, be put on the waiting list. The DHSS targets for the length of waiting lists are one month for urgent cases and one year for non-urgent cases, but these are not always achieved and waiting lists do vary around the country.

Some possible ways you may be able to hurry admission along.
- ▶ Ask whether there is a register of people willing to come into hospital at short notice — where someone cannot accept the booking made. Ask if you can be on this list.
- ▶ Don't provide a long list of dates when you **can't** come into hospital.
- ▶ Ask your GP to contact the hospital on your behalf, if the doctor feels that you have been waiting longer than the average.
- ▶ Ask your GP whether another hospital may have shorter waiting lists. However, you would need to go through the whole process of referral again, at a second hospital.
- ▶ A private hospital **may** have shorter lists. A private consultant cannot get you into an NHS hospital more quickly.

Before you go into hospital, you will almost certainly be sent a booklet, advising you what to bring and giving details of visiting times, etc.

House Officers and **Senior House Officers** are also called house surgeons in departments carrying out operations, and house physicians in medical units. All newly-qualified doctors spend some time as house officers. As a patient in hospital, you are likely to see house officers more frequently than any other grade. If a doctor is needed at once, a house officer will be on call to attend to the emergency.

Anaesthetists belong to a speciality like any other in which doctors can progress to the rank of consultant. As an NHS patient, you cannot specify the particular anaesthetist you wish to see. In most cases, the anaesthetist will visit you before your operation. If you do not see the anaesthetists they will always read your case-notes and discuss your case with the other doctors.

Nurses

The nurse in charge of a ward is called a **Sister** or **Charge Nurse**, where the responsible nurse is a man.

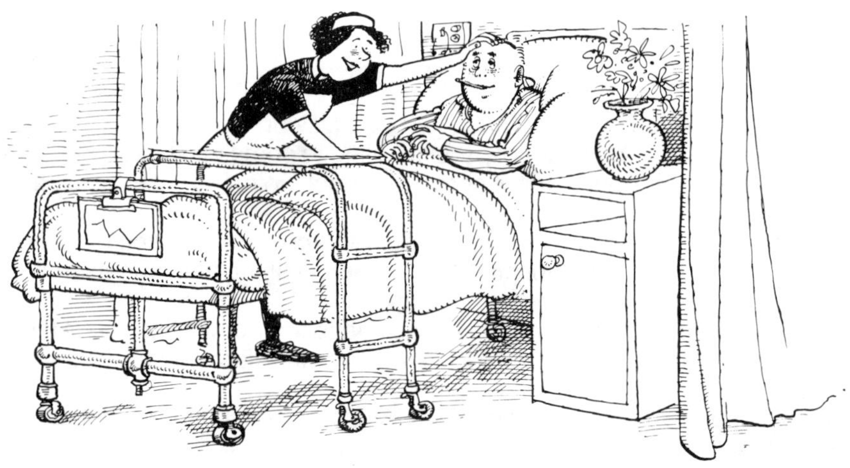

Below the Sister there are **Staff nurses** and students, with the first year students at the bottom of the career ladder. Nurses are either **RGN**, **Registered General Nurse** or **EN(G)**, **Enrolled Nurse (General)**. Enrolled nurses are more practically trained and do not have the theoretical knowledge of RGNs.

Nursing Auxiliaries are care staff who work under the supervision of trained nurses, carrying out practical caring tasks such as bathing and feeding patients. In a **continuing care** ward where old people who are not acutely ill but are too frail to manage independently are nursed, some of the routine care may be given by **nursing auxiliaries**.

Medical Students are attached to each consultant's team in teaching hospitals and occasionally in other hospitals. A group of students may watch while you are examined and a student (under supervision) may conduct an examination. The presence of students is taken for granted in teaching hospitals, but you are entitled to object if you do not want to be examined by them, and your permission should be obtained.

It can be difficult, however, to say how you feel. You may feel awkward about refusing to co-operate with a system which is working for your benefit. An article by Susan Hale, a retired hospital social worker who had found herself on the receiving end of patient care, described how one lady gathered her courage to assert herself in the face of the consultant's teaching round.

"Patients and their relatives often complained 'they never tell you anything do they?' One lady tried to overcome this by making out a long list of questions and reading them aloud to the consultant and his entourage. She ticked off his answers with a red biro pen. Such audacity got sharp looks from the sister and fellow patients held their breath in admiration. I am glad it worked. No-one had the courage to follow her example but I think the consultant was more forthcoming for the rest of the round and the lady herself was triumphant." (*Both Sides of the Counter* by Susan Hale in *New Age*, Spring 1984.)

Radiographers, **Occupational Therapists**, **Physiotherapists**, and **Dieticians** are all registered practitioners whom you may encounter during a stay in hospital.

The **Radiographer** is responsible for taking X-rays, administering radio therapy and carrying out certain other tests, eg. scanning. The doctor or consultant who asked for the tests will have all the details of your case and can explain them for you.

Most **Occupational Therapists** work in rehabilitation units in hospital. Despite all the cartoons and jokes about people in plaster making wickerwork waste-paper baskets, their work is to help people to recover skills in caring for themselves, for example after a stroke or accident. If you are recovering from a stroke or similar illness, an occupational therapist may take you on a home visit to assess the need for any helpful aids and adaptations.

Dieticians, at the request of the doctor, will give you appropriate advice. They may see you in hospital, the out-patients clinic or at home.

Looking to the future

All these hospital staff, and patients as well, can sometimes seem to be the victims of the system — whether the pressure is on the nurses to have all the beds 'done' by 10.30, on house doctors working long hours, or on patients whose needs may not fit in with the routines and expectations of the hospital. What are the possibilities for change? A major report looks to the future.

One of the most significant changes in recent years has been the introduction of 'The Nursing Process'. This is a system of care which is designed to suit the individual needs of the patient. A very full case history is taken and a plan for the patient's care is worked out, involving all the staff concerned.

As consumers of health care, how can we make our wishes known and help to improve the quality of our health service?

One way is by not being **too** impressed by all the new technological advances and by the wonder drugs which have wiped out so many of the killer diseases of the past.

A 1984 report from the Royal College of Physicians sounds a note of warning:

"When the National Health Service was established, few drugs were available on prescription. Today, there is a vast range. This pharmaceutical revolution has brought much clinical benefit to patients of all ages, including the elderly for whom both quality and expectation of life have been improved. However, these improvements have been 'bought' at the expense of an increased incidence of adverse effect and iatrogenic* illness, particularly in older people."

Older people have more drugs prescribed for them than do younger ones; and this is not simply because older people suffer from more disability and disease. There is a real problem with repeat prescriptions which are issued over lengthy periods for older people who may have difficulty in getting to their doctors' surgeries. Not only do older people take more drugs, but they are more likely to suffer adverse reactions to them.

How can we help ourselves?

Campaign for drugs to be supplied with labels giving simple, clear and easily read instructions about their use.

Make sure that we are not guilty of hoarding drugs, of taking drugs prescribed for someone else or for ourselves for some previous ailment. Burn or flush down the toilet any medicine that is not finished up during a period of illness.

Make sure that we **ask** about side-effects and mention any other tablets being taken at the same time, particularly drugs bought over the counter at a chemist's shop.

We can also try to ensure that the feelings, opinions and needs of older people are represented in the general voice of public opinion. It's not just a matter of grumbling and muttering in the privacy of our own living room. Do think about getting involved in campaigning for attention to be paid to the services older people need — whether it is screening facilities for the early detection of disease or more attention to be paid to the problem of over-prescription of drugs for older people.

Patient participation groups began with the idea of letting the consumer's voice be heard alongside the professional's.

Patient participation is based on the idea that co-operation between patients and the medical profession will help to improve the services and the facilities in general practice and at health centres.

The first patient participation group (PPG) was formed in 1972 in Oxfordshire. There are now about 40 active PPGs throughout the country who make up the National Association of Patient Participation.

The main aim of patient participation is to provide a time and place for patients, doctors, health visitors, therapists and other medical workers in the community to come together to discuss issues of common concern

---

* *'iatrogenic'* means 'caused by medical treatment.'

and interest. By becoming involved, patients have found that they are able to influence doctors and other health workers, to the benefit of the practice as a whole.

For further information about setting up and running a patient participation group at your health centre write to:

Mrs Joan Mant
Chair of the National Association for Patient Participation
Hazelbank
Peaslake
Guildford, Surrey GU5 9RJ

We talked to one older lady about her experience of a group. Mary Stapleton became involved in the Centre Users Group at her local health centre in central London 9 years ago. She joined as a representative of a local voluntary agency, but stayed on as a private member after her retirement.

The group has accomplished a good deal since it began, promoting health education activities and also 'fun events' at the centre. "We want to see it really used as a health centre, not an illness centre", she says. They want to expand their activities, running health courses in the afternoons and have published several editions of a **centre users guide** which has proved very useful.

Mary says that belonging to the group has made a great deal of difference to her personal life:

"I've learned a great deal and I feel I now have a group of friendly doctors to turn to whom I can trust, should I ever need their help. Other members of the group have become close friends and it's become the centre of my social life."

The Community Health Councils or Local Health Councils

The CHCs were set up in 1973, in order to ensure that patients' interests in the NHS were represented effectively. The members of your local

Community Health Council are appointed by the local council, as delegates of local voluntary organisations and community groups, and by the Regional Health Authority. There are over 200 CHCs who came together in the Association of Community Health Councils for England and Wales. The equivalent organisations in Scotland are called **Local Health Councils** and in Northern Ireland they are **District Committees for the Health and Personal Social Services**.

Each Council or Committee has a local office with a member of staff available to deal with enquiries from the general public.

What do the health councils do?

The Health Councils act as watchdogs. They send observers to Area Health Authority meetings, where they have the right to speak, but not to vote. This enables the local CHC to keep up to date with what is happening and to convey local people's views to the Health Authority or Health Board.

CHCs and local health councils provide consumers with information on local health care, such as chiropody services, NHS dentists, voluntary groups as well as details of the National Health Service. They may visit local hospitals and report on the standard of services. They may support and promote health courses and conduct surveys and produce local reports. Councils vary, however, and some are much more active than others.

Your Health Council can advise you how to set about making a complaint and tell you to whom it should be addressed. Typical issues that people have felt the need to complain about include such topics as ill-fitting dentures, delay in obtaining medical treatment for a stroke victim, and a GP not coming to visit a patient later found to be seriously ill. The Council cannot take any action itself with regard to individual complaints.

The Health Councils are only as effective as the strength of local support. So if you have a good idea or a grumble about the National Health Service encourage your health council to campaign to ensure that our health services are developed around the needs of local people.

You can find the address of your local Health Council by writing to:

Association of CHCs of England and Wales
Mark Lemon Suite
Barclays Bank Chambers
254 Seven Sisters Road
London N4 2HZ
Tel: 01–272 5459

The Association of District Committees
for the Health and Personal Social Services
Northern Ireland
27 Adelaide Street
Belfast BT2 8FH
Tel: 0232 224431

or to

The Association of Scottish Local Health Councils
21 Torpichen Street
Edinburgh EH3 8HX
Tel: 031–229 2344

Other sources of help

So far, we have looked at the services provided by health authorities. But much of the help people receive in their own homes comes from social services employees, rather than from health workers.

Social Services Departments (in Scotland **Social Work Departments**) are local government offices administered by the local authority. They have responsibility for a range of services which can be of crucial importance to older people. Social Services have four main areas of responsibility.

▶ Providing services to enable people to live at home, eg. home helps, meals-on-wheels, lunch clubs and day centres, laundry service, aids and adaptations in the home.
▶ Staffing and running residential accommodation and supervising private and voluntary old people's homes.

▶ Employing qualified social workers, who will be able to help and advise clients and liaise with other agencies and individuals who can provide support.

▶ Making information on services available, not only the statutory services, but also information about the range of private and voluntary help in existence.

Services at home

The list of services available to people who need help to live independently in their own homes is a long one:

Home helps
Services for the blind, deaf and physically handicapped
Night-sitting service
Laundry facilities
Day care in a day-care centre
Loan of nursing equipment, eg. commode
Recuperative holidays and respite care
Occupational therapy
Physiotherapy
Meals-on-wheels
Telephone installation and rental
Supply and licence of television
Transport to day-care
Home adaptations and loan of aids, eg. wheelchair

Unfortunately, there is a wide variation in the provision of these services. Meals-on-wheels, for example, are available on 5 days a week in some areas, in others on 2 or 3 days and, in a few places, on 7 days per week.

You can get access to these services through a social worker. Too often, older people are at the end of the queue when it comes to skilled social work help. With the recent attention paid to child abuse and other dramatic problems, older people are sometimes neglected, or passed on to less skilled or experienced staff. Luckily, this is not always the case and many social workers find work with older people particularly rewarding.

"It can be an opportunity to work with an exceptionally interesting group of adults: those who have adapted to enormous change and coped with total upheaval of their lives; and who may need a little help to go on living the lives they, in the most part, enjoy and want to continue to enjoy."*

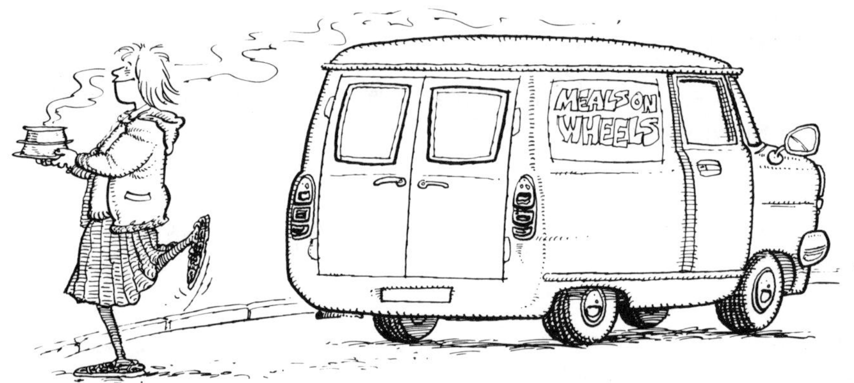

Don't be afraid to contact your local service and ask for a visit from a social worker.

If you have the main responsibility for the care of someone who is very frail, perhaps a husband or wife or a sister or brother, the burden of this can become almost intolerable as you yourself grow older. A social worker can help you practically, as well as lending a sympathetic ear. Respite care, usually in a residential home, can be arranged for your relative, giving you a vital break.

Social workers do not only advise on the statutory services available from local and central government agencies but will also advise on help available from voluntary organisations. Quite often, a paid worker with your local Age Concern or Old People's Welfare Association will be based in a Social Services department and staff of the Citizens' Advice Bureaux also work closely with Social Services.

---

* Mary Marshall, *Social Work with Old People*, Macmillan Press.

The DHSS

The Department of Health and Social Security is sometimes confused with Social Services, because of the similarity of the names. The DHSS is the authority responsible for your state retirement pension and supplementary pension, if you are eligible for this.

This is not an appropriate place to go into detail on pensions and allowances, but we can recommend two excellent booklets, which will help you sort out your entitlement:

Your Rights, published each year by Age Concern, and available from them at Bernard Sunley House, 60 Pitcairn Road, Mitcham, Surrey.

Your Pension, now in its 31st edition and available from Pensioners' Voice, 91 Preston New Road, Blackburn BB2 6BD.

There are all sorts of allowances available for help with particular problems — for instance, if you are cared for at home by a younger relative, he or she may be able to receive **attendance allowance** or help with fuel bills. Similarly, if you have difficulty in getting about, you can receive **mobility allowance** up to the age of 75, provided you apply and qualify for it before your 65th birthday.

You do not need to visit your local Social Security office in order to get advice and help on sorting out your entitlement on pensions, etc. A Social Security Officer will visit you at home if you are unable to get to the office.

If money worries are affecting your morale and well-being, do look for help. As well as the local DHSS office itself, you can get sympathetic advice from your local Citizens' Advice Bureau. Another source of advice on social security matters is:

The Money Advice Centre
The Birmingham Settlement
318 Summer Lane
Birmingham 19

Do enclose a sae if you write for help.

Help the Aged also publishes a range of free information leaflets, including one on Welfare Rights.

Write to:

> Information Desk
> Help the Aged
> St James's Walk
> London EC1R 0BE

or telephone the advice 'Hotline': Tel: 01–250 3399.

Help with housing

Having a safe, comfortable home is essential for a healthy, independent old age. Where can you get help if your home is neither safe nor comfortable?

If you are a council tenant . . .

. . . and are worried because your home needs repairs, you can get help. Councils have a legal duty to keep their property in good order. Your first step should be to go and see your Housing Department and/or the Environmental Health Officer. Always follow up your visit with a letter and keep a copy.

Some council tenants can now apply for grants to improve their homes. You need the Council's permission beforehand or you will not be able to recover the money you spend. You should not embark on improvements yourself without professional advice.

Sheltered housing with a warden on the premises is part of the housing stock of many local authorities. You can apply for a transfer to this sort of housing.

Another alternative is to apply for a transfer, either directly to the Council to move to another property it owns or through a **mutual exchange** with another tenant in the kind of housing you need. You may also ask your Council to nominate you to a **Housing Association** owning flats or sheltered accommodation suitable for retired people.

Many housing agencies and local authorities are now building 'very sheltered housing' which comes mid-way between a residential home and the independence of a sheltered flat. This 'extra care' solution makes it possible for residents to stay in their own flats, rather than face a move to residential care or hospital.

If you own your own home

If your home lacks facilities or is in poor repair, grants are available for such repairs as:

▶ installing bath or shower or inside toilet;
▶ dealing with damp or poor insulation;
▶ rewiring or installing central heating;
▶ major work on roof, floors or walls.

Grants for improvements only cover part of the cost (usually between 50 and 75 per cent) but you may be able to raise the balance through a **maturity loan**. This uses your property as security and you pay only the interest, with the loan being recovered from your estate when you die. If you are on Supplementary Pension, the DHSS will provide the interest payments.

If you are a house owner, you may be able to sell up and buy into a private sheltered housing scheme. For further information contact:

The National Federation of Housing Associations
30–32 Southampton Street
London WC2E 7HE.

Another source of help with housing problems is:

SHAC (The Housing Aid Centre)
189a Old Brompton Road
London SW5 0AR

who publish numerous booklets on aspects of housing legislation and policy.

Your local **Housing Aid** or **Housing Advice Centre** can also help. You can find their addresses from your Town Hall or local library. Local councillors also have a wide knowledge of local conditions and housing problems. Ask how to contact yours at the Council Offices or Citizens'

Advice Bureau.

It may be, however, that you are feeling that you can no longer cope independently and that the time has come to think of a move into residential care. What is available?

Residential Homes

Part III of The National Assistance Act of 1948 (part IV in Scotland) required local authorities to provide residential accommodation in homes for elderly people who required care and attention and had no-one to provide this. The earliest homes developed from the old poor law institutions and inevitably some of the bad reputation was carried over. People's fears about 'going into the workhouse' still lingered.

People who live in local authority residential homes are expected to pay for their maintenance according to their means, up to a certain limit. If a resident has no more than her basic pension, she is expected to surrender most of it for her keep, being left only with a small amount for personal expenses. The type of accommodation offered in the homes, eg. single or shared bedroom, is not affected by whether the resident pays the full cost or pays only a part of her state pension.

Residents in homes are now both older and much more frail than they were a generation ago. Community support services have made it possible for people to live independently at home much longer than in the past, at the same time as there has been a large increase in the numbers of the very old. Homes have changed too, making use of aids such as bathing hoists and lavatory adaptations and often offering extra care for the more physically dependent residents.

Private and voluntary homes

Approximately a fifth of the places in residential homes in Britain are provided by the private and voluntary sectors. The care provided in these homes includes both the best and the worst available in this country.

The supervision of private and voluntary homes is the responsibility of social services departments or social work departments and your local department will be able to provide a list of registered homes. In recent years there has been a great increase in the numbers of private homes, reflecting the growing demand, particularly in areas such as the coastal districts of Wales and the South. This trend has been strengthened by an increase in the number of cases in which the fees of private homes are met out of Supplementary Benefit,* in situations where a place in a local authority home is not available.

For information about residential homes in your area, contact your social services or social work department. There are also national lists and directories, which you can consult if you are thinking of a home in a different part of the country — perhaps near relatives or friends.

One such list can be obtained from:

The Elderly Accommodation Council
1 Durwood House
31 Kensington Court
London W8 7BH
Tel: 01–937 8709

Two useful publications are:

A Buyer's Guide to Sheltered Housing published by Age Concern and National Housing Town and Planning Councils and the *Which? Guide to Residential Homes* produced by The Consumer's Association, 14 Buckingham Street, London WC2 N6DS.

---

* situation will change in April 1988.

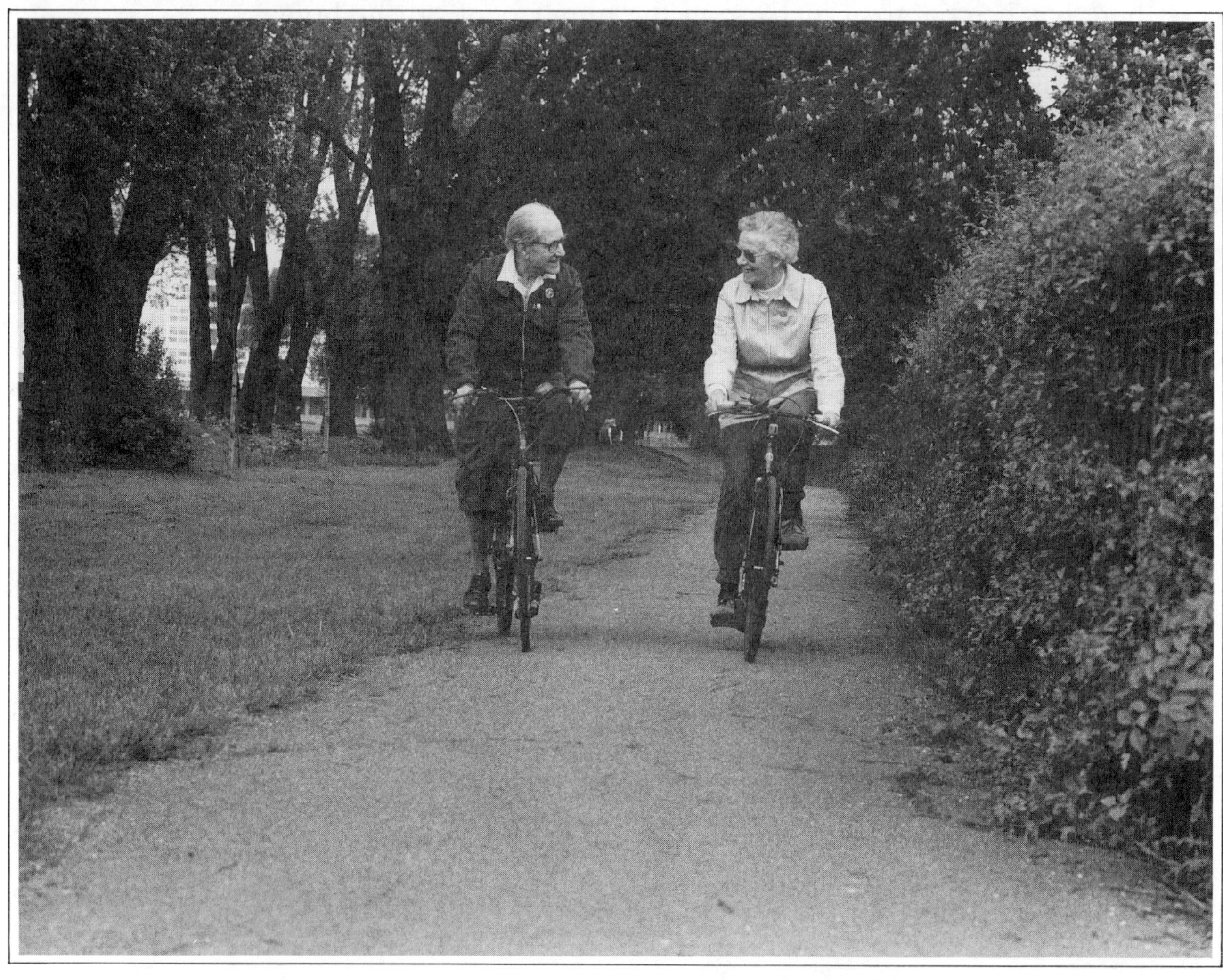

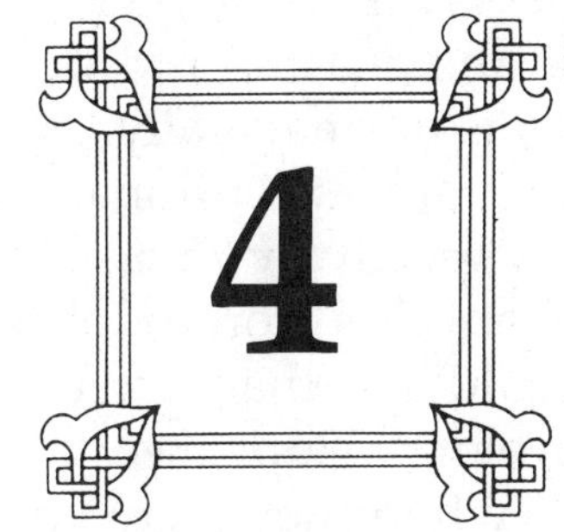

4

MOBILITY: GOING OUT AND STAYING IN

Mrs Tweed is 80 years old and describes herself as in good health for her age:

"Well, I should say if you can get up each morning and have your food and then knock about a bit and do little jobs and perhaps walk out, I should say that was normal really."

Although there are exceptional cases like Tom Young and Arthur Wright who, at respectively 75 and 70, spent three weeks in the summer of 1986 cycling from Brighton to John O'Groats on antique bicycles, most older people would say that, for them, ageing involves slowing down. The majority of older people we talked to felt that they now lived at a slower pace than when they were younger. This wasn't a source of worry — it was seen as just a normal part of life.

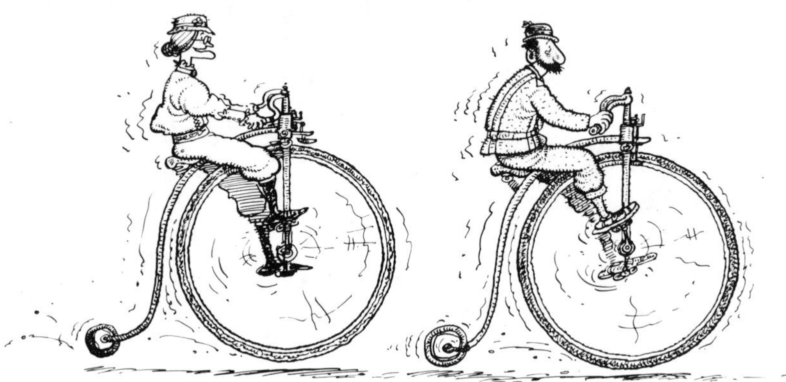

Mrs Hall, who has lived with her daughter's family for the past year, told us what this means to her, when she talked about the daily routine in the house:

"It's murder in the morning, John has to be out by a quarter to eight and the bus picks up Frances [her handicapped granddaughter] at quarter past. My daughter whizzes about getting her dressed and ready and chasing the others to get off to school. I just make sure I stay out of everyone's way!"

Mrs Hall has no wish to be caught up in the exhausting hurly-burly of workaday life. Her role as grandmother gives her the chance to choose her own pace, steering clear of the rush, but able to help out where she is needed. Most older people would agree with her that the freedom to choose one's own pace is one of the real benefits of retiring from work. In this chapter we look at staying active and mobile, having a good quality of life, but slower.

A fresh look at life indoors

We looked in *Chapter One* at some of the physical changes that take place as you grow older. Some of these, such as changes in eyesight, might make it more likely that you will have an accident at home, unless you take action to cut down the risk.

Every year in Britain about three million accidents occur in people's homes — accidents which are serious enough to be treated in hospital or by a doctor. Falls are by far the most common accident for people over 65. A great many of these accidents could have been prevented, if people were willing to look carefully at dangers in their own homes and make the necessary changes.

Ask yourself these four questions:

1 **Can you move about your home easily?**
Can you rearrange your furniture and other effects to help keep areas of movement free from clutter? Don't try and move heavy things by yourself. Ask a friend, neighbour, relative or local volunteer or Community Centre if they can help if you want to shift anything heavy. Check your home for trailing leads. Can you rearrange your appliances to relocate trailing wires out of harm's way?

2 **Could the lighting in your home be better?**
Failing sight and poor lighting combine to increase the risk of falls. Good lighting on landing, stairs and by the bed is a worthwhile investment.

3 **Is your floor an obstacle course?**
Check around your home for frayed and curly edges and holes that could trip you up. Watch out for spills and greasy patches in front of the kitchen sink, by the cooker and near the pet's food bowl.

4 **Can you reach?**
Can you reach shelves, cupboards, windows or door catches that are

in daily use without straining? If you have to store things out of reach, **never** stand on a stool. Should you think about investing in a step-stool if you reach to high cupboards or shelves frequently? Alternatively, have a look at your storage space; can you rearrange some items to make things in daily use more accessible?

If you take a long look at your home now and are concerned to make it more suitable for your needs as you grow older, then help is available to make adaptations and improvements.

The first question is 'Who is going to pay for it?' If you are a registered disabled person or on a low income you may be entitled to quite a range of benefits and concessions. Thousands of people every year do not claim benefits to which they are entitled. The way to establish your entitlement is to ask to be assessed by your local DHSS office. Start by getting the leaflet *Which Benefit?* from your DHSS office which summarises all the benefits. The Age Concern book *Your Rights* is a good starting-point too, and it may pay you to go and have a chat first with the people in your local Age Concern office.

Another line of approach is to ask to speak to an occupational therapist at your local social services department (in England) or social work department (in Scotland). She may be able to help or advise you about aids and adaptations in the home such as bathroom and toilet rails, raised seats and other aids. If you, or someone you live with, are severely disabled you are entitled to receive help with aids and adaptations to your home and you should ask to be assessed.

The Disabled Living Foundation will also give you friendly and helpful advice on every conceivable aid and adaptation in the home, from simple tin-openers suitable for arthritic fingers to sophisticated conversion units to help people in wheelchairs. They do not sell aids themselves but you can go and see a variety of aids on show at their Aids Centres. You can make appointments for individuals and for groups. It's always helpful to see and discuss aids and adaptations before buying. Contact the Disabled Living Foundation, 380–384 Harrow Road, London W9 2HU or The Scottish Council on Disability, Princes House, 5 Shandwick Place, Edinburgh EH2 4RG.

Housing Trusts and Building Societies

If you are an owner occupier and considering some fairly major altera-tions to your home such as modernising your kitchen or putting in central heating, the Anchor Housing Trust have produced a very useful directory of local sources of financial help, practical assistance and advice on repairs and adaptations for elderly people in their own homes. It is called *Staying Put in Retirement* and is available from:

Age Concern Information Department   or from   Age Concern Scotland
60 Pitcairn Road   33 Castle Street
Mitcham   Edinburgh
Surrey CR4 3LL   EH2 3DN

The Anchor Housing Trust in co-operation with the Abbey National Building Society have been piloting a scheme for older home owners of loan finance for improvements such as putting in downstairs bathrooms and lavatories and stairlifts. The way having been paved, a number of building societies have indicated a willingness to approve interest only loans.

"I am 65 years of age and in spite of arthritis I get about as much as possible. I have recently had central heating installed and my kitchen modernised with the help of the Anchor Housing Trust who have helped me to get an interest only loan on the house from the Abbey National. I am grateful to have my own home and garden and to live in a pleasant road with good neighbours."

This kind of financial arrangement is one which you will need to consider very carefully and perhaps get advice on, but as a general rule it is a viable option particularly for older house owners who live alone.

Out and about

A fresh, positive look at your home is an excellent starting-point, but most people recognise how important it is to be able to go out and about.

"I make a point of going out every day, even if it's only to the newsagent at the corner. If I didn't get out, I feel it would be easy to let things slide. It helps me keep up my standard."

What if getting out of the house is a major problem?

For many people, like Miss Jones, who wrote to us, home can sometimes seem like a prison.

"I do try not to let it get me down, but sometimes I feel very weary of these four walls. My nephew sometimes takes me out in his car, but it's such a performance! I feel so frustrated by not being able to walk without my frame and him to prop me up."

Many day centres all over the country own specially adapted minibuses which can be used to help people like Miss Jones get out and about. Your local Age Concern office will be able to tell you what is available. Help the Aged has provided more than 240 minibuses to projects helping elderly people all over the country. There may well be one near you.

There is also an organisation called **Contact** which runs a network of groups of volunteers and elderly people who get together regularly for tea in the home of a volunteer hostess, the volunteers using their own cars to provide transport. If you want to know if there is a group in your area, write to:

Paul Freeman
Contact
15 Henrietta Street
Covent Garden
London WC2E 8QH
Tel: 01–240 0630

who can provide information on groups all over Britain.

Walking

It is a sad fact that people on foot in our towns are at greater risk than those driving about in motor vehicles. Walking is nearly as dangerous as riding a bike, from the point of view of the accident risk, and far more dangerous than being a passenger in a car.

37% of those killed in road accidents are pedestrians and it is older people who are most at risk. Pedestrians over 70 have 5 times the rate of accidents of young people in the 25–39 age group.

How can you take care of yourself?

The answer is not to stay indoors, but to take active and sensible precautions when you go out. The kerb drill we all learned as children, 'Look right, look left, look right again, and if all clear, walk straight across' is no longer taught. Children are instead encouraged to 'Keep watching and listening all the time'. It is good advice for all ages, now that there is a far greater number of vehicles on the road, travelling at greater speed.

You can also lend your support to local campaigns to make the roads less dangerous to pedestrians. Cars parked on pavements, damaged paving stones, very short sequences on crossings, all make walking about the town unnecessarily stressful. Many pensioner groups are already working to publicise these dangers and you can become involved in this sort of campaign.

You can also make sure that, if you wear glasses or use a hearing-aid, you wear them when you are out and about.

Public transport

Older people are less likely than younger ones to have cars, and travelling on buses and trains can be a problem. With buses, a whole list of difficulties can arise, from actually getting to the bus-stop, waiting in a queue, negotiating automatic doors and high steps, to reading the destination and reaching bells and handrails inside the bus. Some local authorities are far more aware than others of the special needs of older people. For instance, special 'kneeling' buses with a platform which can be lowered to help you get on and off the bus are in service in some areas. Again, there is a place for pensioner groups to get involved, making sure their voices are heard among the planners.

Trains are probably easier and more popular than buses. There are many special rates available to older people, not only in this country, but on trains in Europe. A train journey also provides an opportunity to meet new people: men and women who, at home, would be shy of talking to strangers, chat easily to fellow train passengers and friendships can start from these small beginnings.

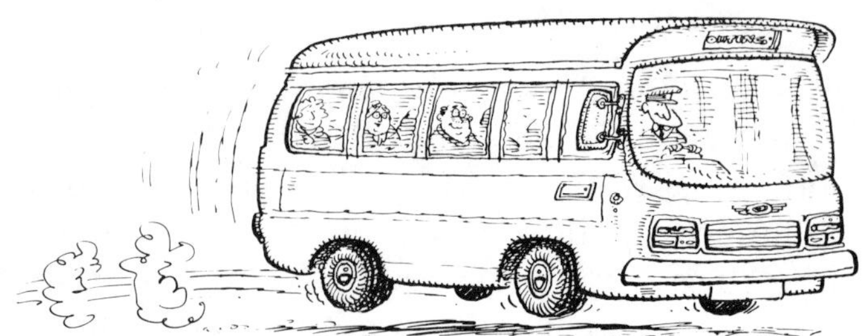

Air travel

Many British people have relatives and friends in Australia, New Zealand, the United States and Canada. Often retired people plan to visit their relatives, once they are no longer working full-time or perhaps when a lump-sum pension is available. Even if you have never flown before, you shouldn't be put off air travel by worries about your age.

British Airways run 'Reunion Clubs' for families whose relatives are abroad and hundreds of people, some very old, take these special flights every year. There are obviously some medical conditions which make flying inadvisable and, if you are having treatment, you should consult your doctor about your plans.

However, if you are in good health, the airlines probably offer the best service of any of the transport organisations: from wheelchair access and escort services to special diets.

Some tips for air travel

▶ Wear suitable clothes for the weather conditions in the country to which you are going;

▶ If possible, plan to arrive in the early evening, when you can go straight to bed;

▶ To avoid swollen feet and ankles, take little walks in the plane;

▶ Avoid alcohol, which causes dehydration, and drink extra soft drinks — these are often supplied free of charge;

▶ If you are taking any medicine, be sure to carry it in your hand baggage, rather than risk being separated from your luggage.

Two useful publications on transport:
Door to Door: a guide to transport for disabled people is available free from
the Department of Transport. Write to:

Door to Door Guide
FREEPOST
Victoria Road
South Ruislip
Middlesex HA4 0NZ

A free factsheet on travel concessions for older people can be obtained
from:

The Information & Policy Department
Age Concern England
60 Pitcairn Road
Mitcham
Surrey CR4 3LL

or from

Age Concern Scotland
33 Castle Street
Edinburgh EH2 3DH

Please enclose a stamped addressed envelope.

Exercise

Many older people we spoke to mentioned 'taking exercise' as an
important part of looking after their health. This ranged from the very
gentle:

"I try to walk every day, even if it is only possible to do so slowly and a
short way",

to quite a tough programme:

"I am a walker. I cycle and swim and I do a regular routine of exercises each morning."

Unfortunately, although many fit and active people report the good effects of exercise, there are also some widespread myths about exercise and ageing which prevent people having a go. Do you ever find yourself using these excuses?

"Not at my age"

Inactivity is bad for you at any age. You have only to think of how weak and frail you feel after a few days in bed to realise the truth of this.

It is true that you may feel that you do things more slowly than you did when you were younger and that you may notice a loss in strength and stamina, but there is no reason at all why you should not continue to help yourself to keep fit and keep in shape at any age. The more exercise you do the fitter you will feel. The fitter you become the more you will be able to do, and the more you will want to do. One of the symptoms of a lack of fitness is lethargy, so you will need to make that initial effort to get yourself going. If you have grown used to thinking of yourself as an 'old person' you may have gradually been doing less and less for no reason. Little and often is the key, and this is preferable to over-exerting yourself, especially if you have not been taking enough physical exercise for a long time.

"I'm disabled" or "I suffer from a disease that makes it impossible"

If you have been struck by a severe illness such as a severe stroke or have suffered a heart attack, or perhaps have had a serious operation you will know that the first step to recovery is exercise. In hospital, you will have been helped by a physiotherapist to begin gentle exercise.

Whatever your disability or ailment your body needs exercise to function properly. If you haven't taken much exercise for years, take it gently to start with and slowly build up to more strenuous activities.

If you are under medical attention or treatment and if you are uncertain about the sort of exercises that are suitable for you in your circumstances, please tell your doctor or health visitor that you want to try and take more exercise and suggest an activity that appeals to you.

"It won't make any difference at my age"

If you have been fit all your life, the worst possible thing to do is to stop taking exercise when you retire. To be really fit in retirement you will have to earn that rest in your armchair.

It is often easier for most women because the normal everyday housework and shopping keep you moving. The only trouble is that even if you actively enjoy housework, it can get tedious and monotonous and so housework alone doesn't provide the same stimulus as doing something physically active that you really enjoy.

There are often movement and exercise classes designed specially for older people run by local authorities. Often, these are in the afternoon and so are more suitable for retired people.

EXTEND is one organisation which offers special classes for retired and disabled people to improve fitness through movement to music. You can find out about a class near you by writing to:

Mrs Penny Copple
Extend
The Boulevard
Sheringham
Norfolk NR26 8LJ
Tel: 0263 822479

or write to:

The Scottish Extend Organiser
Pam Scott Watson
Tich Gryanach
1 Thornhill Road
Forres
Morayshire IV36 0LW
Tel: 0309 72971

Here are some gentle exercises which were developed for older people by The East Midlands Keep Fit Association. They are suitable for everyday use, and can be started without risk.

Wrists & Hands

To maintain mobility in fingers and wrist joints.
1 Rub hands together. Massage the fingers and wrists. Gently shake the hands. This will bring blood to the area, warming it and make the hands more pliable.
2 Make a fist, then spread the hand and fingers wide. Repeat several times. Spread the hands flat on a table, spreading the fingers wide. Hold a few seconds, then shake hands. Repeat several times.
3 On a hard surface, 5-finger exercises across and back. Single hand first and then both hands together. Shake hands when muscles ache. Later try in the air.
4 Fingers relaxed, rotate wrist several times clockwise. Shake hand and repeat anti-clockwise. Repeat with other hand. Later try both hands together.
5 Sitting on chair with feet flat on floor, slightly apart. With hand relaxed drop it palm down on thigh; lift and drop back of hand on thigh. Repeat several times, taking care to see the elbow is free to move easily. Try each hand separately and later both together.

Elbows, Shoulders, Neck & Head

To relax tense muscles in shoulders and neck which often cause headaches.
1 Standing or sitting on a chair, with arms hanging easily downwards at sides. Lift shoulders up to ears and allow them to drop. Repeat.
2 Same position as No.1. Shoulder circling backwards. Each shoulder separately and then both together.
3 Sitting or standing with feet apart. Drop head forward, roll slowly in a circle to the left, finishing in front, head down. Press neck backwards to lift head slowly. Repeat rolling in circle to the right.
4 Sitting hands on knees, shoulders and elbows easy. Turn head sideways to look over right shoulder. Then turn to look over left. Repeat these movements. Rest and repeat again.
5 Sitting tall on chair. Lift both arms slightly sideways, turn insides of arms to face front, and pull backwards; relax arms so they drop to sides. Repeat several times.

Feet & Ankles

To strengthen feet and leg muscles.
For maximum benefit these exercises should be done barefoot or in stockinged feet.

1 Sitting on front half of chair, holding two front corners for support. Sole of foot brushing the floor forward and backward several times. Repeat with other foot. Allow foot to be easy and loose.
2 Position as in No.1. Lift heel as high as possible and lower. Several times with each foot, then both together.
3 Tap floor lightly with toe, lift foot and tap lightly with heel. Repeat several times with each foot.
4 Sitting on chair with heel resting on another chair or stool. Keep heel on the spot and circle big toe, outwards and round trying to increase size of the circle. Repeat with other foot. Both heels resting on stool or chair, slightly apart. Circle both big toes inwards towards each other, increasing size of circle.

Knee & Hip Joint.

Lifting and lowering body weight to chair or floor, travelling on the floor, sitting or lying

The following exercise will help to maintain or improve the range of these joints and the power of the muscles.
1 Sitting on front half of chair, holding two front corners for support. Lift knee as high as possible, then return foot to floor. Repeat with the other knee. Repeat these movements several times.
2 Pick one foot off the floor, move leg outwards to place foot on floor at side of chair. Lift and return it to the other one. Repeat several times lifting leg as high and as far to side as possible. Repeat with other leg.
3 Sitting sideways on chair, grip chair back with one hand and front corner of seat with the other one. Feet on floor, one foot slightly in front of the other. Lift both feet off floor at the same time, then return them to the floor. It helps to lean backwards with the body when lifting and forwards slightly when lowering. Gradually increase this lean so that weight goes on to feet each time, and from this rhythmic movement it is easy to stand, steadying the balance with the hand on the chair back.

Yoga

Yoga classes are among the most popular courses available at adult education centres. There is no age-barrier to taking up Yoga and many older people report that it helps them relax and improves posture and breathing.

Yoga means 'oneness' and stems from the belief that mental peace, health and physical strength are wholly interlinked. This 'oneness' and predisposition to good health is achieved by meditation, relaxation, breathing and posture exercises. The series of postures practised are generally known as 'Hatha Yoga'. There is evidence to suggest that Yoga helps you control your body functions and can help physical complaints which are caused by stress.

Two correspondents, who came to Yoga late in life, told us of its effect on them:

"I attend Yoga classes at the local school, and through them I've attended one or two lectures on alternative medicine, herbalism, massage, healing and reflexology. I find Yoga a great help when I cannot sleep."

"I have trained to be a Yoga remedial teacher through the Yoga for Health Foundation. I am thoroughly convinced of its value, particularly of proper breathing for the maintenance of health at any age!"

The Yoga for Health Foundation mentioned here is a registered charity. They have an association and nationwide membership linked to Yoga for Health clubs and remedial instructors. They also run a residential centre which you can visit for a day, a week or longer if you wish. Whilst they do not offer courses specifically for older people, there is no age limit and many of their active members are in their 70s and 80s. For further details of the Foundation, its centre and directory of clubs and instructors write to:

The Yoga for Health Foundation
Ickwell Bury
Biggleswade SG18 9EF
Tel: 0767 26271

You may also find classes at your local adult education institute, community centre and natural health centres. Your local library is usually the best place to find out, but classes in Yoga are very popular and you will need to apply early.

Although it is possible to get going on a programme of exercise by yourself, it is a lot easier and more fun to do in a group.

One example of just how much can be achieved is to be found in North Staffordshire. The Beth Johnson Foundation is a local Charitable Trust which has set up a wide range of activities for older people, including an advice service on starting exercise, diet or relaxation programmes.

You can contact them at:

The Beth Johnson Foundation
Parkfield House
64 Princes Road
Hartshill
Stoke on Trent ST4 7JL
Tel: 0782 44036

There is a growing understanding of the benefits for people of all ages of staying active and fit.

You can get help and advice from:

The Sports Council
16 Upper Woburn Place
London WC1H 0QP

or

The Scottish Sports Council
1/3 St Colme Street
Edinburgh EH3 6AA

You probably know someone who has been fit and active all their life and will claim that this is due to regular exercise. The 'experts' are now saying what such people have always known to be true, that 'if you don't use it, you lose it'.

If you are willing to make a start on an exercise programme, there is a great deal of help and advice available now.

Gardens and gardening: activity outdoors and in

Gardening is the most popular spare-time activity in Britain. But for many older people, keeping the garden in good order can become a major worry. Again, the main idea is to choose your own pace. You don't have to be superfit before you start to think about gardening and it's a very rewarding way to get the daily relaxation and exercise your body needs, especially if you are recovering from an illness or managing a disability. The great advantage in gardening is that you can take it as gently or as energetically as you like. It needn't even be an outdoor activity. Some indoor pots or a window-box can provide an interesting hobby and a splash of colour in your home.

"There's not a pair of legs so thin, there's not a head so thick,
There's not a hand so weak and white, nor yet a heart so sick,
But it cannot find a needful job that's crying to be done,
For the glory of the Garden glorifieth every one."

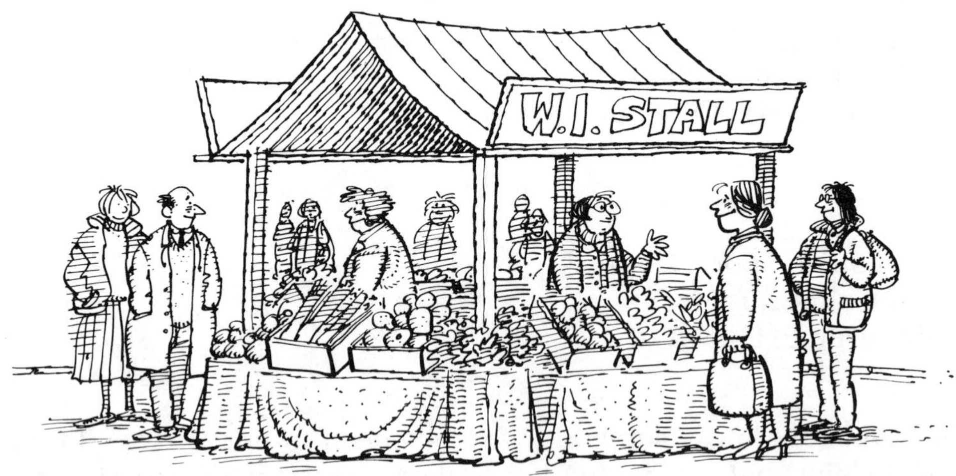

Apart from providing you with a relaxing way to get some physical exercise, it's one practical way in which you can improve your immediate environment, by growing things around you.

Herbs are a good idea because you can grow them on a sunny window-sill or window-box and they don't take up much room and are easily managed in pots and tubs. The ordinary culinary varieties like mint and thyme and rosemary and sage are rich in vitamins and minerals as well as bringing a smell and a taste of the country.

Don't be put off if you have never been keen on gardening and don't know where to start. Your library is full of gardening books and armchair gardening is a very enjoyable way to start, especially in the winter months. One idea is to join a local gardening club. Gardeners are always keen to teach and learn from each other. Many clubs have visiting speakers and 'swop shops' and a range of outings to gardens open to the public. Gardening need not be an expensive hobby. Swapping plants and cuttings is half the fun. For many people their garden is the source of a little business as well: selling plants through such outlets as the Women's Institute markets or raising money for various appeals and charities.

The Disabled Living Foundation (DLF) in close liaison with The Society for Horticultural Therapy runs a gardening advice service for disabled people. This includes advice on design of your garden and the range of tools now available, for instance to help with gardening from a wheel-chair. The DLF also have demonstration gardens at Syon Park in Brentford, Battersea Park and at the Royal Horticultural Society Gardens at Wisley. The DLF also provide a lecture service for clubs. So if you are interested contact:

The Disabled Living Foundation   or   Scottish Council on Disability
380/384 Harrow Road   Princes House
London W9 2HU   5 Shandwick Place
Tel: 01–289 6111   Edinburgh EH2 4RG
                                                                      Tel: 031–229 8632

Gardens aren't just for gardeners either; parks, gardens, little bits of green and trees do more to lift the spirits and sense of well-being than almost anything else. The National Gardens Scheme in aid of the Queen's Institute of District Nursing publishes a little book listing 1200 gardens in England and Wales open to the public.

Write to:

The National Gardens Scheme
57 Lower Belgrave Street
London SW1V 0LR

or for Scottish addresses to:

Scotland's Garden Scheme
31 Castle Terrace
Edinburgh EH1 2EL

Going on learning

In *Chapter Two* we mentioned 'learning something new' as an important way to combat loneliness in your life. Keeping your brain active is as important as physical exercise, if you want to continue to lead an independent and satisfying life. Yet very many older people decide that education is not for them. Here are some reasons they might give.

▶ education is a middle-class occupation for the 'educated';
▶ adult education classes are too expensive on a pension;
▶ education is a once and for all activity for children;
▶ education was a bad experience at school;
▶ education is vocational and has no real purpose in retirement;
▶ adult education is not accessible to people who are disabled or handicapped;
▶ adult education is not a suitable pursuit if you are underconfident about trying something new on your own.

But there is another point of view to consider.

▶ Learning in later life is for everyone. As an older person you bring your own knowlege and experience which is as valuable as any 'formal' education;
▶ The majority of adult education classes have concessionary rates for pensioners;
▶ Learning is a life-long pursuit. Learning is enriched in later life because you are not 'empty vessels to be filled with knowledge'. You

can bring your own knowledge and experience to make adult education a three-way process between you, the tutor, and the other members of the class;

▶ Some people will remember school as a period of discipline and fact cramming. Learning in later life is so much more than the accumulation of facts and the assimilation of information. The object of education at any age should be to fire the imagination and provide you with food for thought and ideas for action;

▶ Education at any age is a way of opening up opportunities, new channels and interests for you. Opportunities to exercise the mind are just as important as physical exercise is to the body;

▶ There is a range of opportunities for people who are visually handicapped, hard of hearing or have problems of mobility that make attending an adult education class seem difficult. In some parts of the country there is an Educational Guidance Service which can arrange courses for house-bound people in some areas. A free list of Educational Guidance Services is published by The Advisory Council for Adult and Continuing Education (ACACE), 19b, De Montford Street, Leicester LE1 7GE;

▶ Taking up opportunities to learn in later life can give a tremendous boost to self-confidence.

If you have weighed up the arguments on both sides and are willing to have a go, how do you make a start?

Where to go

The best place to start is your local **institute of adult education** or **community college**.

Many **polytechnics** run courses specifically designed for learning in later life. These courses are designed to help people who have not studied anything since they left school, and subjects range from creative writing to environmental studies. The Open College of the North West, the Polytechnic of North London, the Middlesex Polytechnic and Hatfield Polytechnic are just a few of the colleges who have run courses specifically for older learners. Many universities and polytechnics also run an open system where you may go and sit in on lectures alongside the students.

One useful guide to Adult Education and training opportunities is *Second Chances*, published by the Great Ouse Press in association with SHE magazine. You will find a copy of this in your local reference library.

U3A Groups

The French talk of retirement as the 'Third Age'. The 'first' age being childhood and youth; the 'second' age being employment and raising a family; and the 'third' age is an active and independent retirement. A University of the Third Age, known as U3A is rapidly growing as a national self-help movement for learning and teaching by and for people in the 'third' age. Local U3A groups have developed out of groups of older people coming together in an *ad hoc* way with common interests. These groups are often linked to local further education colleges or adult education institutes. For further details of U3A and its local branches write to:

Dianne Norton   or   University of the Third Age
University of the Third Age (U3A)   32 Calder Road
6 Parkside Gardens   Edinburgh EH11 3PD
London SW19 5EY

FREE

Dianne Norton also acts as the co-ordinator of FREE which is an association of people interested in promoting a Forum for the Rights of Elderly People to Education. FREE acts as a clearing-house for information on any and every activity or idea that will promote opportunities for learning in later life. They will also help you to set up local and regional learning groups, if they do not exist.

For further information about FREE write to:

Dianne Norton
Bernard Sunley House
60 Pitcairn Road
Mitcham

Surrey CR4 3LL
Tel: 01–640 5431

You can also write to:

The Open University in Scotland   or   Scottish Community Education
60 Melville Street   Council
Edinburgh EH3 7HF   Athol House
Tel: 031–226 3851   Canning Street
                                                            Edinburgh EH3 8EG
                                                            Tel: 031–229 2433

Teaching and Learning

The unique aspect of education in later life is that it offers opportunities to teach at the same time as learning; to give of yourself as well as to learn from others.

Oral History

Nowhere is this two-way process of teaching and learning more evident than in the current surge of interest in living memory as local and social history. Older people are finding that their memories and recalled experiences are much in demand, not only by social historians but by local history societies, local museums, schools and colleges, not to mention television companies and radio stations. Many local history societies and reminiscence groups have published their memories and many groups are affiliated to the Federation of Worker Writers and Community Publishers.

The Oral History Society is the main organisation co-ordinating and publicising work in oral history. For further details write to:

The Oral History Society
Department of Sociology
University of Essex
Wivenhoe Park
Colchester CO4 3SQ

History in your own home

Have a rummage through that old box full of memories you keep in the attic or the cupboard under the stairs. Look through the objects and cuttings and photographs you've been meaning to sort out for years. Ask yourself why you keep them. What memories do they bring back for you?

Sometimes the silliest things trigger off the most vivid memories. They are all part of your life, part of you, as you were and as you are now.

If you want to, share your thoughts with a grandchild or younger person you know or mention it to a friend or group of friends. You might like to go on and start your own reminiscence group perhaps with a view to publishing or making your information available to a local school or museum. You might find it helpful to choose a common theme, such as where you used to work, life on the street where you lived, life at home.

For details of your local oral history, reminiscence or local history group ask at your library or adult education institute. You will also find details of classes from:

The British Association for Local History
The Mill Manager's House
Cromford Mill, Cromford
Matlock, Derbyshire DE4 3RQ

Help the Aged has produced a series of slide/tape programmes called **Recall** which covers the last 80 years in sounds and pictures. This series has been used extensively as a 'starter kit' for groups and a resource for discussions and talks. Interestingly **Recall** is also used by occupational therapists and others in therapy and rehabilitation programmes with older people. Winslow Press also publish a wide range of reminiscence materials.

Help the Aged Education Department has pioneered work in this field because they feel it is very important to try and create situations in which older people can recall, reflect and pass on the benefit of their knowledge and experience in a useful way to others. The concept of exploring living memory with younger people in schools, in colleges and in the local community is one really important way in which older people make a real and valued comment on society, which with the benefit of hindsight, as an older person, **only you** can make.

For further details of **Recall** write to:

Help the Aged Education and   or   Winslow Press
Research Department   Telford Road
PO Box 460   Bicester
St James's Walk   Oxon OX6 0TS
London EC1R 0BE

Ideas for action

So far, throughout this book, we have made suggestions about actions you might like to take to improve your health or to cope with a problem. They won't all apply to you, but one or two may seem sensible ideas for reorganisation. You can select one and concentrate on that, or else make a long-term plan. Here is a reminder of some of our ideas:

SELF HEALTH	CONTACTS
Think before you drink	Health Education Authority Scottish Health Education Group
Give up smoking	ASH (Action on Smoking for Health)
Daily exercise (keep it varied)	Keep Fit Association
Regular physical activity or hobby	Local gardening club; community centre; sports centre; library
Promote the idea of keep-fit classes in your area	Health Centre; Adult Education Inst; Sports Centre; Keep Fit Association; Extend
Take up Yoga or relaxation exercises if you need to find an alternative to control the effects of stress or control your smoking and drinking habits	Adult Education Institute; local library; Yoga for Health Foundation.
BE PREPARED	
Prepare for the loss of a partner or close relative. Share responsibilities and skills, eg. learn to drive, mend a fuse.	Age Concern
Make a will	Talk to your partner

HEALTH CARE Keep your appointments with	Optician Dentist Chiropodist Audiologist GP Therapist
Take exercises if you need to control stress incontinence	GP/Physiotherapist Disabled Living Foundation
DIET Look for/initiate course on food and diet	Health Education Officer (ask at your Health Centre) Community Health Council Adult Education Institute
Check your emergency food store. Replenish it from time to time. Always remember 'a little of everything and not too much of anything'.	
ARE YOU WAITING? If you are on a long hospital waiting list, can you move to another list?	College of Health 2 Marylebone Road London NW1 4DX
HOME MANAGEMENT Check your first aid kit. Keep a list of useful addresses by the phone. If you have a disability find out about aids and adaptations.	Town Hall, Occupational Therapist, Social Work Department, Disabled Living Foundation; Age Concern. Scottish Council on Disability.
Think about your drug routine and management Clear out old drugs hoarded.	Local pharmacist
TAKE ACTION Take a course in first aid/resuscitation Grow something (even if it's just a pip in a pot).	St John Ambulance or Red Cross

SELF-HELP

Contact a self-help group that meets your needs	College of Health has 1200 contact addresses
Campaign for pensioners' rights issues that concern you most, eg. more health education for older people at local level, better labelling on drugs.	Local pensioners group Plain English Campaign
Seek help if you want to find an alternative to your drug therapy.	'Release' and other self-help groups. College of Health
Look for/initiate a course on alternative therapies	Adult Education Institute Natural Health Centre
Join or start an oral history/reminiscence group.	Adult Education Institute Local Museum Local History Group School PTA
Volunteer. Find an opportunity to give of yourself.	Library, CAB, Age Concern, Hospital, Local Charity.
Try something new. Take a risk	Adult Education classes Local travel agent

Set yourself your own targets that suit you best.

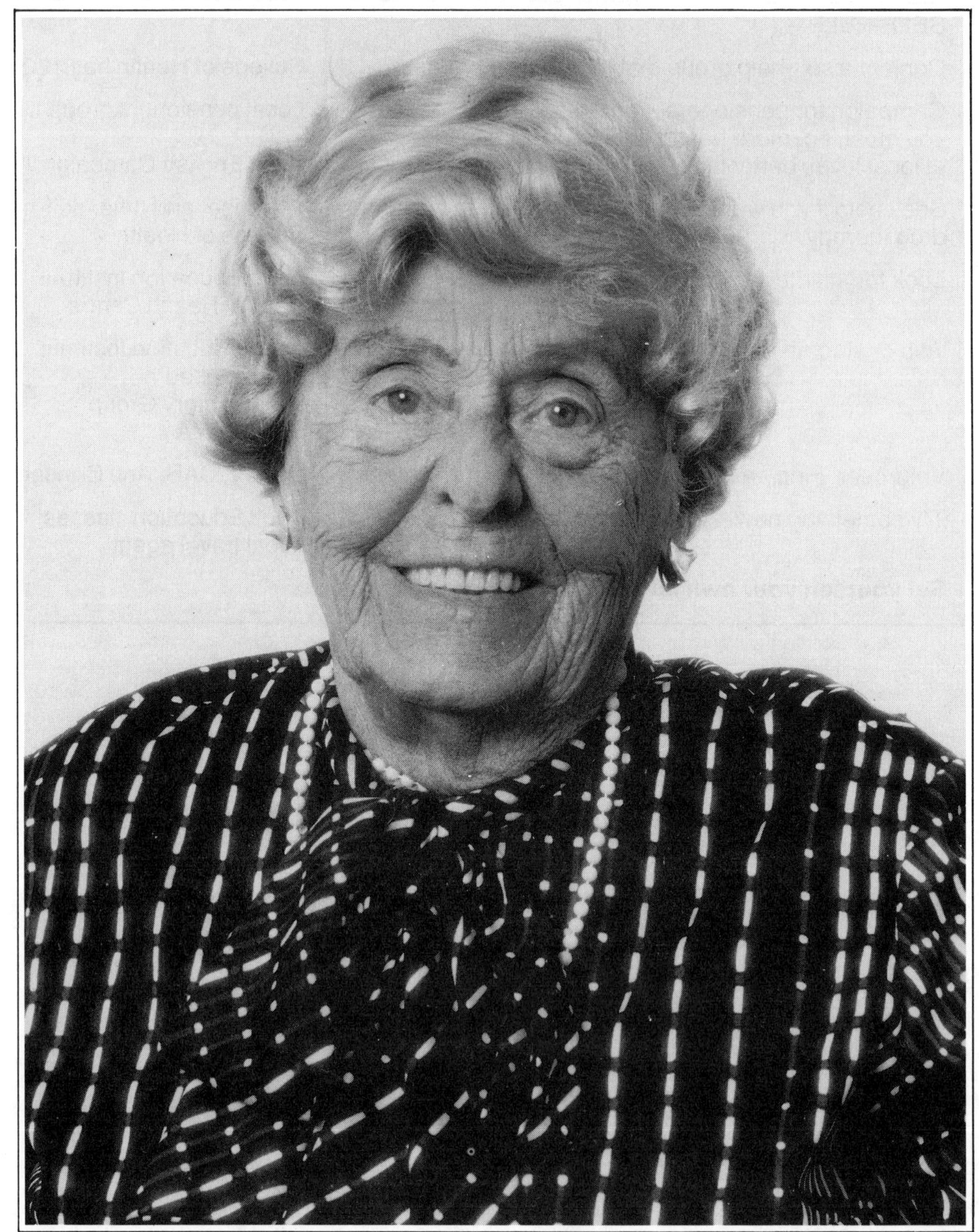

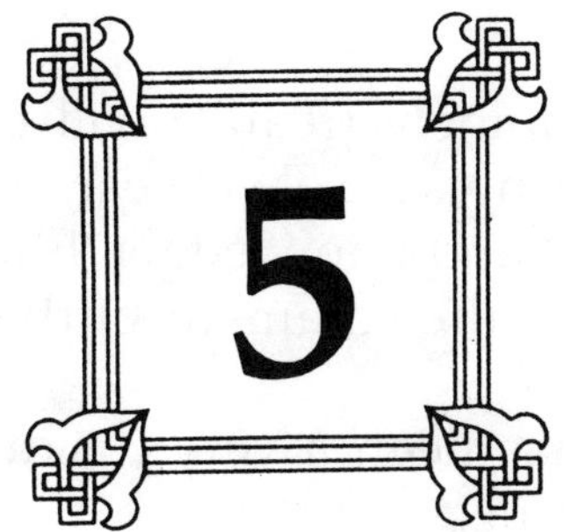

VERY SENIOR CITIZENS — JUST FOR YOU

Dorothy Moriarty

(Please note:
Dorothy Moriarty is writing from her own personal experiences.)

Introduction

I hope that my homely treatise will find readers among the really old, because I am old myself. Two years off a hundred which gives me the authority of first-hand knowledge. 'She knows what she's talking about', will, hopefully, be the comment of the 80s and 90s, on my practical and intimate realism.

Growing old has been a very insidious and gradual process where I, myself, am concerned.

In my seventies, though ostensibly living in my son's house, I continued to pursue my own life, in my own way. Taking on temporary jobs as cook-housekeeper; deputy Mum while Mum and Dad went off on a second honeymoon. Masterminding, and cooking, luncheons and dinner parties. I took on anything and everything with a brassy confidence that sometimes led to near-disaster! Or that is how it seems to me when I look back. But there was always a laugh at the end of the day.

I carried on into my eighty-second year, when arthritis struck. Quite suddenly, as I was crossing a busy road, my right leg gave way and it was agony to move it. But I was lucky in my doctor. An X-ray and her diagnosis put me into circulation in no time at all.

Restrictions on standing about cooking made me look for another avenue to explore. Baby-sitting.

I became a surrogate Granny, and I never lacked employment. Then, in my odd moments, I wrote and had published a short story or article. I even won the odd competition. Also, twice a year I visited the American half of my family in the USA. At 98 I still do this, with the help of wheelchairs and caring people.

I am not very mobile now, but my trusty cane, and exercises for my wobbly legs, keep me on the move — though public transport is out of the question.

And now I have ended up in a wonderful Home for the Aged. Here I am learning a new way of life, new values, new interests; making new friends while keeping up with those I have left behind. And every morning I tell myself "One day at a time". Then I look round my cosy room, with its view of a flower-bright garden, and I add: "Count your Blessings, Honey."

Just for you

Old people (ie. my generation), do not usually ask for advice; they prefer to give it.

And yet, looking at my contemporaries, or near-contemporaries, for I am 98, I am aware that advice is what many of us need.

Advice on how to live courageously, happily, peaceably and graciously. Detailed advice about changing attitudes and about changed human relationships; about substitute interests — in a word, learning to adapt before loving Grandma or Auntie becomes real hard work for the family. What I have to say may be useful for distracted relatives to help the OAP on their conscience and, perhaps, on their doorstep. It may help, because we do sometimes listen to our own generation. Being something of a feminist I deal only with the problems of women who are growing old, who have barricaded themselves behind a closed mind. Basically I am considering the problems of the over-80s. By then, living will have become more difficult. When you have little money left in your account it becomes important to spend it wisely; and in that respect your remaining years can be compared to money in a bank.

This chapter is written with the idea of gingering up the lives of old people by one who knows, because she is old herself. By one who has experience of the frustrations, the diminished effort at decision-making. At ninety-eight I can certainly claim to speak with authority on the subject.

But, for those who have given up, perhaps through no fault of their own, those who have drifted beyond the point of no-recall, there is only one solution, the dutiful daughter, or the home with nursing care. And I am thinking, as I write, not of the well-off senior citizen, the ones who can smooth the wrinkles out of life with money; nor of those who still share life with a partner. No, I am considering the case of those who, like myself, can just get by, with care.

Those who save-to-spend, whose 'mad money' is the result of sensible planning.

I give advice to the old, the lonely, the bored, because I have managed to avoid these things and believe I can now help others to a satisfactory solution.

I write for the people who 'can't be bothered' which is the danger point for the ageing, if they but knew it.

My chapter deals with adaptation; adapting to a new way of living; a new set of interests. All the problems created by learning to adapt, ie. accept.

Saving energy

When one is over eighty the saving of energy is very important. You will discover that you have just a daily quota of once unlimited energy. So use it very very carefully. Here is a simple example of what I mean. When I go to church I sit all through the service. Bobbing up and down takes more out of you than you realise. Sit wherever you can on whatever will bear your weight. I have even perched on one of those big metal cigarette ash-stands.

But saving energy does not mean dropping off to sleep at intervals throughout the day, for this will mean a restless night.

Try not to use sleeping-pills for even the milder ones become a habit just through suggestion. Get one of those 'sleep button' radios and turn it on to background music loudness; this will mask all the little annoying and disturbing household noises that may make sleep difficult. Counting sheep, a glass of beer or a boring book are other sleep inducers.

When you go out, take a walking stick. Not only does it act as a lever to take the strain off stiff legs, much as the pole in the hands of a pole-vault contestant, it is also a safeguard against a fall — and old bones are brittle.

And do try to train your head to save your legs. So, if your bedroom is upstairs, have a bag of some sort into which you can put such items as glasses, a pen, a notebook, your current novel, to save you going up and down stairs — constructive thinking, in fact.

And, for shopping, use one of those little trolleys. It is not good for an old person to stagger along carrying heavy shopping bags. I know that a trolley in a bus is a nuisance but it is a real and necessary one. One is apt to say, 'I am only going to buy one or two small items so I won't take the trolley.' Wishful thinking.

You will see things on the shelves of your supermarket that you had forgotten you needed.

Adjusting to surroundings

1. Living in the family home

This is the ideal of course because it should ensure your being wrapped in an atmosphere of loving and caring. But it has its snags.

Be very sure of how the situation can be handled before you burn your boats. If there is even a latent antagonism lurking in your mind think again. I know an old lady who lost her husband after fifty years of marriage. She panicked! She sold her house, left all her friends behind and went to live with her widowed son and his family. His wife had died a few years earlier and his three teenage children had grown up free to run their lives and the house-keeping to their own ideas. They bitterly resented the intrusion into their privacy of a grandmother they scarcely knew.

The result was disaster; and the unfortunate son (a busy consultant doctor), was pig-in-the-middle of these warring personalities.

The Americans cope with this situation by converting the basement of their house into what they call 'an in-law apartment'. We had a neighbour whose in-laws came to live with their family. They had an upstairs three-room apartment that opened onto a landing.

The unfortunate daughter-in-law once said to me, "My mother-in-law is a lovely person, but she drives me nuts. Every time my telephone rings or someone knocks at the front door, she pops out like a cuckoo from a clock."

So keep yourself to yourself. Lead your own life. Insist on paying a rent. Be self-sufficient. Ensure this with a small roaster-toaster oven, and electric ring that can double as a grill; a mini fridge, an electric kettle, your own television. Then you are all set for a contented life.

2. *A Shelter Home*

Here there will be a Warden to keep a motherly eye on all who are under her roof. Remember she has to keep to the rules and she may not be warm enough or clever enough to bend these without losing her job. So do not expect special treatment. If she is the tight-lipped fussy sort, keep out of her way and never voice your complaints. Mischief makers are always to be found in places like this. If you must grumble do so to those of your visitors who live in Timbuctoo or other far-away places! The trouble about being one of a community like this is, of course, the 'popper-in'. Try evasive methods first, even if you resort to putting a hat on your head; "I'm so sorry, I'm just going out". Issue the occasional definite invitation and neighbourliness can be kept on that level. The same advice applies if you live in a small house in a long row of similar houses. 'Poppers-in' are a problem we senior citizens have to deal with wherever we are. But reflect, without all these trivial problems life would be dull indeed.

3. *Living in your own small house*

Neighbours are really important here. Even if you have to sacrifice some of your privacy. Old people are very vulnerable to neighbourly advice. Have a Judas eye let into your front door. Don't open your door to strangers. Always ask to see credentials. Beware of conmen; and even beware of small boys. Don't you recall the story of the kind old lady who opened her door to a tearful small boy and followed him into the garden to look for a mythical puppy? So his pals were able to get in and snatch this and that. We are always being admonished, yet friendly snoopy neighbours are our best safeguard.

Living alone; long dark winter nights with little niggling fears coming and going in your sub-conscious. So why not do a bit of conversion and find a suitable tenant? It's certainly worth consideration.

4. *Living in an Institutional Home*

Living in a Home with nursing care is the final test of ability to adapt to change. The very thought of life in an institution scares a lot of people. Don't let it scare you.

Once again I speak with authority and first-hand knowledge for I am now a resident in just such a home.

It has to be run on institutional lines but the atmosphere is that of a home from home. There are nearly a hundred of us here and the great majority have some kind of crippling disability. I, myself, hobble around with a trusty cane.

Living in a home like this demands diplomacy. Never get too involved with any one person; never allow yourself to grumble aloud. Don't hold aloof from others; and join in communal activities when possible. Keep a low profile and don't stir up petty jealousies. Never take sides, but, on the other hand, don't allow yourself to feel priggish like the Pharisees of old.

Make friends, but keep to a relaxing privacy. Visits to your room by invitation only.

Yes, I know it is tough to break away from family and home. But you have become too much of a responsibility to them. You need more care than you, yourself, realise.

It's not fair to a modern family coping with modern stresses and tensions.

So — go while the going's good and God Bless.

Keeping up appearances

Have you got into the habit of trailing around most of the morning in slippers and a dressing-gown?

Very bad for your morale. Meet each day with a confidence that is built up by the effort of washing, dressing, make-up, and don't complain "I can't manage my hair these days". Go out and buy a wig. It saves money because hairdressing prices have risen too steeply for the likes of you and me to afford them. A wig means one less chore in the morning and the knowledge that you can look your neighbour in the face without self-consciousness.

And do get it into your head that 'old' and 'ugly' are not synonymous. When I was ninety I was asked to a party to meet a local VIP. I put on my best wig, a treasured and well-tended two-piece, a dust of powder, a touch of lipstick, and yes, a whiff of lavender water.

At our introduction he came towards me, hands outstretched and a sudden smile on his face. "Why, you're beautiful", he told me.

You see, having been informed of my age, he expected to be confronted by a Witch of Endor, no less.

I am not beautiful any more but I do use all the 'props' suitable and helpful in creating at least a pleasant impression on the people around.

Then, when I go to bed I put my dental 'bridge' into a tumbler, my wig on a stand, wash the make-up from my wrinkled face, and hope there will be no night emergency to rob my image of its glamour.

Clothes

How can we, the pensioners, afford even the 'special offers'? The answer is Jumble Sales. Cast-off garments, yes, but many of them hardly worn at all. A Jumble Sale, especially one sponsored by a church with a well-off congregation, can be very rewarding. And Jumble Sales are fun. Try and head the queue even if you have to wait for an hour or so before the doors open. Take a tape measure with you and do be careful to keep an eye on any garment you may have put down while you measure or try on. I turned round at one sale to see my own coat being looked over by a prospective buyer.

Then there are the 'Nearly New' little boutiques. But these days their prices have risen noticeably.

I am one of the lucky ones. I am an annuitant of RUKBA, The Royal United Kingdom Beneficient Association.*

Twice a year I can ask them for clothes or 'soft furnishings'. And the clothes they send me are superb. The ladies of the clothing department are fairy godmothers waving wands over us OAP Cinderellas.

Annuitants who may read this will confirm my words.

* RUKBA helps elderly people from a professional and similar background on very low incomes, primarily with financial support. For more information write to the Director, RUKBA, 6 Avonmore Road, London, W15 8RL

Make-up

An ageing skin does need what I would describe as a delaying action cream. A cream rubbed sparingly into withering cheeks night and morning. Eyebrows tend to vanish with age, so an eyebrow pencil is a must. Use it with a light hand because beetling black brows are not a feminine asset.

Lipstick? Yes, but not too red, as this would emphasize sunken and sallow cheeks.

And what about those insidious little hairs that mar the femininity we should cherish and preserve? A tube of hair depilatory cream, put on three times a week, is the answer to that problem.

But do resign yourself to the stark fact that when youth has gone it has gone beyond recall and do not attempt to snatch it back with the help of boxes and pots filled with false promises.

I remember vividly an occasion when I accepted an invitation for a make-up session in one of Kensington's big stores. I was in my seventies and the illusion of being a 'good-looker' still lingered in my mind. I went up to London, entered the store, showed my invitation card and a synthetically beautiful young woman took me in hand. She worked on my elderly face for about a quarter of an hour; then she handed me a mirror and stood back to admire her work.

"Does Madam look even sixty?", she asked a colleague.

"Fifty, not a day over fifty," the colleague assured her through iridescent lips.

I left the shop and made for my train home, well pleased with what I had seen in the mirror. I was going to a bridge party that afternoon. The train I thought I should be boarding at Waterloo was waiting at the platform.

I showed my ticket to the polite Pakistani collector at the gate. "No, no, Old Lady," he told me; "wrong platform. Old Lady's train at No.3."

Well, I got the message. I wiped off that lying make-up before I went to my bridge party. All the same, don't go to the other extreme. Don't ever say, "Make-up? I can't be bothered, not at my age."

And don't be too proud to ask the girl at the cosmetic counter for advice. She probably has a granny who needs just simple basics, like you.

Pets

Pets can complicate life for the old. Unless you live in your own house a dog or cat can be the reason why doors may be shut in your face. 'No Pets' is a clause in many leases and lettings.

So, if you must have a pet it will have to be something small; a bird, perhaps? A canary, a parrot, a budgie?

Or you might revert to the small furry animals of your youth, a small tank of tropical fish or a goldfish in a bowl? These moving specks of rainbow colours can even have a therapeutic effect pyschologists assure us. I know my dentist has quite a big tank of tropical fish in his waiting room.

There is no doubt, though, that pets are not only a responsibility, but a tie. You get 'flu', a cold or a touch of lumbago and the cleaning out of a bird cage seems more than you can tackle. So do be very sure that you need a pet before you take one into your life.

Substitute interests

You are coming up to, let us say, eighty. You are increasingly aware that walking and stooping are becoming more and more of an effort: so the time has come for adjustment. To find interests that require the minimum of physical effort, yet which can be a good substitute for those you have to give up.

For example: you have always been a keen gardener but now find that even the long-handled tools the family gave last Christmas are not the answer. So what? The answer is window-boxes and house-plants.

But before you rush off to buy the plants go to your local library and get a couple of books on the subject. Then you won't put an African Violet to wither on a sunny window-sill or a cactus to sulk to nothing in a dark corner.

We have all heard of people who chat to their plants and claim that they get some kind of response. Who am I to doubt?

For if I have some disbelief in this excessive claim, I am in no doubt at all about the companionship one gets from plants.

And they demand so little in return. Some, indeed, seem to thrive on neglect. The philadendron, for instance, is almost impossible to kill. It goes on for ever climbing up a stick or hanging down in lovely green loops of foliage.

The Spider plant developing its dangling family at the end of stems like dried straws, is another survivor.

So is the Maranta or Rabbit Foot. Fascinating with its imprints of dark green with pale green edges that never seem to curl up and wither. These three indestructibles should make good starters for your indoor garden. These house-plants plus a few others should make a good substitute interest for you if you live in a flat or a bed-sitter. But if it is a case of your living in a house with a small garden where the weeds are taking over, look for a neighbour who would be glad of an 'allotment' in which to grow vegetables and perhaps, flowers. We had a neighbour who did just that and both parties got great satisfaction from the arrangement. You can arrange a nominal rent and a share in the vegetables as they come to maturity. If you have not already got an outside tap, get one fixed up to avoid the friction of your rent-a-garden friend having to fill his watercan up at your kitchen sink.

And the occasional gardening chat will give pleasure to both of you. But don't overdo it. He has come to work, not to talk. Old people have to beware of garrulity.

Sport

So you were quite a star in the local Tennis Club when you were young, and even someone to reckon with in your fifties.

And badminton? You were good at that too.

So what will you substitute now that you can no longer run and jump and volley?

Search around and don't be too choosy.

Croquet? Clock golf? Swimming perhaps. Swimming is a wonderfully adaptable sport. And how about bingo, when you can no longer go to the races? And if you are house-bound, how about those wonderful electronic games? Don't close your mind to suggestions.

New and Acquired Interests

These unlike substitute interests are those that have to be developed from scratch. Many people have retired from demanding jobs that left no time for the arts and crafts.

Not to worry. Think back to what you liked doing in kindergarten. Think of Grandmother Moses and recall the praise you got long ago for your 'primitives'. What she could do, you, at least can attempt. So go out and buy brushes, watercolour paints and cartridge paper. If you only end up as a painter of greetings cards for the family you have accomplished something and ensured the passing of many pleasant hours.

Your adult education college will have art classes and if you can get to these it will put you in touch with people and ideas.

Photography is another subject for consideration as a serious hobby. Sharpen your wits all the time; it is so easy to sink into apathy crying, "Too late, too late", like the White Rabbit.

I had a friend who worked for her degree in literature, and graduated at seventy-two. She deserved the bottle of champagne produced by her family. And her face was scarred from the injuries received in a car accident a few months before she graduated. But she was not put off by that painful interruption to study!

And what about that pen set the family gave you for Christmas? Why not put it to good use and find yourself a penfriend? Let the postman's knock be something to which you can look forward. Once you get the knack of writing letters the words will trickle from your pen. Even the humblest letter-writer contributes to history. And truth, far from lying at the bottom of a well, is often found in a bundle of old letters.

"All very well", you say, "but my arthritic fingers make it difficult to hold a pen."

No problem! Get a tape recorder and exchange 'live' letters. And still on paper and pen projects, why not have a go at competitions? Get a copy of the *Competitors' Journal* to find out how to go about it.

When I was 89 I was a winner in a nationwide competition. I won a Mediterranean holiday for two.

Write letters to the women's magazines, send them useful household tips. Collect these from friends, from childhood memories and write them down in an exercise book. You may end up acquiring the odd two or three pounds and seeing yourself in print.

I have a friend of ninety who gets days and weeks of fun and employment in baiting bank managers and Inland Revenue officials. She sits in her Baker Street flat at a table strewn with forms, dealing with her own tax problems and those of her sister, who is a ward of court.

Bored? She doesn't know the meaning of the word. Then consider crosswords. People can become addicted to these brain-teasers. For this interest you need a dictionary and a Roget's Thesaurus.

Bird-watching

All you need for this is a pair of binoculars and a window at the back overlooking a garden — any kind of garden — a neglected strip with trees for preference. Also a simple handbook on birds. You are then set up as a very humble member of the great bird-watching community. Watch the birds by day, jot down your findings at night, and you will discover that the hours, like the birds, have wings.

Needlework

If your sight and your fingers are a handicap, and they well may be if you are over eighty, try to get interested in, say, hooked rugs and forget the quilting and the petit point you once found so rewarding. Hooked rugs can be fun and, like a giant jigsaw puzzle, everyone can have a go. I remember a retired colonel in a guest house where I was staying who had us all doing our little bit in the evening when we gathered together in the lounge. The resultant crouching tiger was a masterpiece. And you may be able to knit with those outsize needles you can tuck under your arms, continental fashion.

Games and other pastimes

Cards, Patience, or Solitaire.

Quite absorbing when you're on your own; get hold of a handbook.

There are more than a hundred games of patience to tease and stimulate.

I remember a childhood friend who never missed his nightly game of 'Miss Milligan', one of the more complicated games of patience. "Better than sleeping-pills", he would say as he laid out his miniature cards. "It settles my mind for sure."

Then there are the social get-together games like whist and bridge. Bingo is another collective amusement . . . But don't let it go to your head so that it empties your pocket. Put into your handbag just the amount of money you can afford to lose, so that by this limitation you are prevented from trying to recoup losses.

If you are by nature gregarious, watch out for news of 'outings'. You can enjoy the basic fun of a jollification even if you can no longer scramble amongst rocks or climb up hills. And do not forget to take a folding canvas chair with you for you can no longer collapse gracefully onto the beach or grass.

And don't spoil these things, bingo and outings by being 'snooty'. Remember that 'The Colonel's lady and Judy O'Grady, are sisters under the skin'. All too often I have heard people say: "Outings? Oh, no, they wouldn't be my sort of people, dear."

My greatest friend came from a Yorkshire working-class family and she very often dropped her 'aitches'.

I had a cultured middle-class background. I first met her when she had retired from the prison service in which she rose to deputy governor of Holloway. We would meet two or three times a week and set the world to rights. Two women from totally different backgrounds who came together in a friendship that endured till she died, and beyond. For I still miss her and thank her for all those hours of pleasure.

Travel

Given reasonable health and mobility, don't, as I have already warned you, let conventional hand-outs about being too old for this and that come down like a cloud on your view of far horizons. Reach out to them.

For what is to stop you visiting your daughter in Australia, or your son in the United States? "Too far", they say. "Too cold." Nonsense. Don't be mesmerized into a static old age.

I know that many people are nervous of air travel; but, unless this is a phobia, you can think and talk yourself out of it. That is, if the final objective — such as family reunion, is important to you. Picture all the train crashes, car crashes, and coach crashes. Yet how gaily you board a train, get into a friend's car, and sing on a coach outing.

Also, impress on your nervous sub-conscious the fact that you will be visiting the people who matter most to you — Family.

I practise what I preach; twice a year I visit my family and friends in Boston, Massachusetts: Spring and Autumn. Or should I say 'Fall'?

I was nervous at first, but now, boarding a plane makes me no more jittery than if I were boarding a bus. And living for a few weeks in that different atmosphere is like the re-charging of batteries.

And the journey is less harassing than getting across London by public transport.

Having made my decision I go off to my local travel agent. I choose the one that, like myself, is old and well established.

I pick out an assistant whom I decide will be both caring and practical. I have found me a wonderful girl called Jean, and we have a most satisfactory relationship. I have become her 'special' old lady.

Here is my recipe for easy travel, step by step.

Having arrived at my travel agent's, I seat myself on a stool at the reception desk, opposite Jean.

We plan my journey with an eye to economy as well as comfort. And here, let me point out that this advice is not for the well-off OAP, but for the save-to-spend Senior Citizen like myself, who has to make the most out of a little.

I travel, therefore, on a super APEX ticket, ie. advance payment economy class. Which means that I have to book and pay at least 21 days in advance.

Then Jean and I agree on insurance that settles for all pre-flight medical hazards, and also covers my four weeks' visit to Boston. We then consider seating. Important, because I have some circulatory trouble, like many old people. I must be able to stretch my legs. "Leave it to me", says Jean. "You must have a bulkhead seat so that there are no seats in front of you to cramp your movements. And of course the usual wheelchair will be ready at the airport here and another waiting for you in Boston. I will book your seat 28 days before your flight date; as you know we can't do it earlier. But I and my computer won't forget and your boarding pass with seat number will be here on the office desk for you to pick up."

So much for the preliminaries and when the great day arrives I find everything laid on to save me effort.

I travel on a Sunday, for Heathrow on Saturday is pure bedlam. A courteous elderly gentleman or a chatty, eager student, wheels me along a seemingly endless corridor. On and on, past the queues for passports, a brief halt to show mine. Another short stop where a little black silhouette of a lady is painted on a yellow door.

"Just a moment", I say, getting out of my chair. Because I have never yet discovered whether one may use the toilet on the plane before take-off.

I have childhood memories of notices on long distance trains which instructed one not to use the toilet while the train was stationary. The toilet being just a covered hole, one can understand the reason. But there is modern plumbing on planes, so why do I worry?

Anyway we finally arrive at the departure lounge, where we head the queue. When the gates open, off we go again.

I am first on the plane. I step out of my chair, press a discreet pound into the hand of my charioteer before a stewardess takes me and my flight bag in charge; and so, down the aisle, to my seat.

The flight bag is one of those light canvas affairs that footballers carry around. In it I have my supply of pills. Most old people have some form of daily medication. I don't put them in a case because luggage can get mislaid or lost. I also put in a pair of soft slippers, to ease my feet on the journey.

A pair of 'blinkers' (eye-shade), made out of a strip of black silk and kept in place by an elastic band, is a 'must'. For my bulkhead seat is immediately below the big television screen. This enables me to cat-nap on the outward flight and get some sleep on the return flight which is a night one. And, with the blessing of my doctor, I swallow a couple of mild sleeping-pills. I put a nightgown, toothbrush, etc. in the bag because

I don't want to have to unpack my case when I arrive.

On the outward flight one is given immigration and customs forms to fill in, so have a biro handy.

As for the return journey, Jean and her computer will have arranged all that, but, with the warning, "Prior to your return phone, the airport to confirm everything, at least 72 hours beforehand."

This happy travel picture applies only to those who go to family.

Otherwise — move around, yes, but only within the comforting radius of the NHS. And it's a good idea if you live in the South of England to visit the North and vice versa. It's surprising how little we know of the other half of our country.

And the 'off-peak ticket' and the 'off-peak hotel' are real money stretchers. And incidentally, you'll meet quite a few other Senior Citizens who have kept their spirit of adventure. People who refuse to be labelled 'too old'. The world is still your oyster, and if you failed to find the pearl when you were young, you may yet pick it out with those arthritic fingers.

And finally . . .

A Dangerous Practice

I have come to the conclusion that far too many of my contemporaries have a ridiculous and unreasoning mistrust of banks. They keep their savings stashed away in a teapot, in a biscuit tin, under a mattress, in the potting-shed. By so doing they create a situation that is a positive menace, not only to themselves, but which drags even the wise ones who do use a bank, into the danger zone. Because the petty thief and the conman have come to look on the family of OAPs as potential victims, an easy prey. I sometimes wonder if social workers should not be more insistent in their warnings. The closed mind attitude probably defeats them.

So, please, those of you who read this, and are guilty of stashing away your money, go off to your bank and deposit it, and then do a bit of campaigning amongst your friends who 'don't believe in banks'.

Tell them about your neighbour down the road. Two men with a ladder told her she had loose slates on her roof. She paid them in advance, and they certainly climbed onto the roof; then they disappeared to get non-existent slates. If she had had her money in a bank, that fairy tale would have fallen on deaf ears.

Safety

You must, at all times, be prepared to put safety before dignity. Go downstairs backwards, one hand on the banister rail and one resting on a stair tread. Never mind if you do look like shaggy bear, tell yourself, "Safety before dignity".

Get out of a bus backwards — you can only fall forward a few inches.

In the bathroom

In the bathroom you can still be independent, even if stiff with arthritis. Take your bath towel and drape enough of it along the rim of the bath to give a good grip. Having got into the bath go down on your knees and manoeuvre yourself into position — safe and recumbent. To get out, repeat the towel gripping operation. But if your hands are really contorted with arthritis, resign yourself to operating a shower. Even though we, real 'oldies', do not like showers!

The Snub

I think as we grow older and more dependent, we tend to become resentful of help; resentful to the point of ungraciousness. Refusing to accept the kindly hand held out as we drag our stiffened limbs up from a chair. "No thank you, I am quite well able to manage by myself." A curt and unsmiling refusal.

The Bore

We are apt to talk too much and always about ourselves and our shrunken world, which seems to develop a fresh grievance every day. We should try to listen more, and reach out to the interests and problems of those around us. For enjoyable conversation is give and take. And why not hold out the helping hand yourself sometimes? At the supermarket check-point give up your place in the queue to the harassed young woman with the crying baby and a trolley full of goods. So hand out smiles instead of snubs — grow old graciously.

Tackling the more embarrassing problems

Now we discuss some homely hints that should help you to deal with the unpleasant health problems created by an ageing body.

Most of us find, for instance, that we get up to pass water two or three times during the night. The bathroom may be way down a long dimly-lit passage we dread blundering along on sleep-stiffened limbs. So provide yourself with a quart size plastic jug to replace the old chamber pot you can no longer use. The jug is easy to hold and use standing up: it is quite an efficient urinal. And it's easy to keep clean and to disinfect. If you are going to stay at a friend's house or an hotel just pop it into your case.

Incontinence troubles many old people for muscles get flabby and inefficient. Don't wring your hands and moan. Go out and buy a rubber sheet for your bed. And consult your health visitor or your doctor about wearing one of these modern gadgets of which there are many these days.

Also, weak bladder muscles can be strengthened when you pass water; use a stop-go technique every time.

In this same context, ie. muscle deterioration, the intestines very often need extra stimulation. For one thing are you having three regular meals a day and using roughage in your diet? To keep your intestines moving they need bulk stimulation.

In my youth people used a thing called a 'Japanese medicine ball' to stimulate flabby tums. You may find a modern replacement for this homely gadget.

Chiropody

You will probably need help, literally to keep you on your feet. Bunions, callouses and trimming your nails, especially those that tend to be in-growing, may be very difficult, if not impossible for you to deal with.

So get your NHS chiropodist along. And don't forget to soak your feet in hot water before he arrives.

★   ★   ★

And now, goodnight, fellow pensioners. And, before you climb into your bed, have you remembered to check the shelf above your bed or the table beside your bed?

Your glasses? Your electric torch? Your box of pills, all counted out and ready for the morning? Your bottle of sodamints in case a touch of indigestion should keep you awake?

Right. Turn on your sleep-button radio, pull up the bedclothes and go to sleep.

"Matthew, Mark, Luke and John, Guard the bed that I lie on."

And may all those lovely moments from your past be with you in dreams.